Rapid Weight Loss Hypnosis: Guided Self-Hypnosis& Meditations For Natural Weight Loss & For Effortless Fat Burn& Healthy Habits, Developing Mindfulness & Overcome Emotional Eating

By Meditation Made Effortless

Table of Contents

To the Narrator

The Introduction, Induction, and Deepener should be 45 Min Long

Stop Emotional Eating and Increase Confidence should be 30min long
Reprogram Your Mind for Long Term Health
should be 30 min long
Letting Go of the Weight Protection should be 25 min long
Eat in Moderation should be 20 min long
Find Better Foods should be 20 min long
East Less and Enjoy More should be 20 min long
Do not Eat Junk Food should be 15 min long
Change Your Eating Habits 30 min long
Ego Strengthening Script should be 25 min long
Confidence is the Key should be 25 min long
More Weight Loss should be 25 min long
Change is the Key should be 25 min long
Healthy Lifestyle should be 25 min long
Road to Life should be 30 min long
Low Carb Diet should be 20 min long
Reinforcement Script should be 15 min long
Affirmations should be 180 min long

"…" means take a breath while speaking before you continue.

PAUSE (for a few breaths)

LONGER PAUSE (give time to allow the listener time to imagine what you've suggested

Introduction

Thank you for choosing **Rapid Weight Loss Audio**... This recording contains everything that you need to listen to, to be able to lose weight rapidly.

From eliminating junk food craving, to increase exercise motivation, to boosting metabolism, to loving yourself more to boosting confidence and self-esteem, this ten hour recording will allow you to program your subconscious mind to lose weight much faster. It will tell your subconscious mind for positive physical changes to help you reach your ideal goal weight. To make you look slimmer, leaner, and healthier that will make you ultimately feel happier and confident about yourself.

Pause

So, congratulations on taking this step to listen to this audio that will make you focused and allow you to stick to your weight loss plan. Every time you listen to this audio, you get more and more focused on knowing that you are capable of achieving anything and losing weight just gets easier.

Pause

I would like you to sit or lay comfortably, where you will not be distracted. Do not listen to this audio when your mind requires your conscious attention. You are going to go on a beautiful inner journey where you will day-dream, imagine many positive things, and listen to affirmations that will keep you motivated throughout your weight loss journey.

Pause

Listen to this audio only when you are relaxed and stationary. Please use headphones so that you can focus on the sound of my voice.

Let us start…

Begin recording

Induction

You are now listening to the sound of my voice… and the sound of my voice only …and as you continue to listen to each word I say…you allow yourself to relax more and more.

Pause

I wonder if you could take a deep breath…hold it for a count of 5… and then exhale.

Pause

Let's start now.

Breathe in Deeply…

Pause

Hold for a count of 5

1… 2…3…4…and 5

Now, exhale…

Pause

Once more, take another deep breath…

Breathe in…

Hold for a count of 5 — 1, 2, 3, 4, 5 (slowly)

Now, breathe out…

Pause

Once more, take another deep breath —

Breathe in

Hold for a count of 5 — 1, 2, 3, 4, 5 (slowly)

Now, breathe out

Pause

And, come back to your normal breathing pattern…

Pause

— And, I wonder… if you could simply bring all your focus and attention to the center of your eye-brows…with your eyes closed…try to look at the center of your brows and focus on the point between them…that's right.

Pause

In a moment, I am going to talk to that part of you, which is highly creative…the part that knows exactly how to help you imagine or create anything with the help of your mind's eye.

Pause

And… I know you can do it… because everybody can…we all have a creative mind, that has the ability and capability to create and imagine images in our mind. The same mind that make us draw, daydream, dance, write, and do all the creative things.

I know you must have imagined or visualized or day-dreamed many times in your life. And… our creative part helps us imagine and visualize.

With the help of our creative mind, we can visualize, imagine, write, paint, and dream…and I am going to be talking to that part of you today.

Pause

Your very powerful mind is listening to me and I wonder if it can help you imagine a staircase somewhere that leads you to a hallway with the door at the end.

Pause

Just imagine it and I know you can do it, because everybody can.

It could be a staircase made of stone or wood or metal, it does not matter…what matters is that you notice a staircase with 20 steps. And, as you notice yourself standing on top of it…you can easily notice the hallway just at the bottom of it.

That's right.

Get the knowing of the stairs and the material they are made of…

Pause

You are going to go down the staircase and each step you go down, you feel even more relaxed and drift more and more into a calm state of mind.

So, let's take the first step…

20…put your right foot on the step

19…starting to go down the staircase

18…deeper and deeper

17...drifting down

16...becoming even more relaxed

15...listening to the sound of my voice

14...deeper and deeper

13...focused even more on my words

12...relaxing even more

11...deeper and deeper

10...half way there

9...you can notice the hallway

8...and you wonder what's behind the door

7...relaxing more

6...focused on my voice

5...reaching the hallway soon

4...you can notice the floor and walls of the hallway

3...even deeper

2...about to reach

1...almost there

0...step in the hallway

You are now beautifully relaxed...with your light body, you move forward into the hallway and reach the door.

The door leads you to the deepest part of mind, where what I say will stay there...

It's the deepest part of your mind...that's right...

You are going to open the door to the deepest part of your mind as I count down from 5 down to 0...

5, open the door

4...you are entering the deepest part of your mind

3...the door has opened for you to absorb everything that is important for your highest good

2...its opening now fully

1…its open and you are open to all the suggestions…

That's right…

Pause

Stop Emotional Eating and Increase Confidence

You continue to remain in this deep and focused state of mind and every breath you take and every word you hear allows you to deepen and maintain this wonderful state of relaxation even more.

Pause

Your powerful creative mind is open to all the positive suggestions and every breath you take only means that you are allowing these positive suggestions to sink into your head and heart...

Every breath you inhale... and every breath you exhale takes you twice as deep into this wonderful state of relaxation and opens you up to all the positive suggestions.

Pause

The sound of my voice lets you relax even more and every positive statement that I say moves in every part of your being allowing the new to replace the old that does not serve any purpose...that's right.

Pause

Your conscious mind rests and takes a back seat and enjoys the subconscious mind to be in charge. And your subconscious mind reviews as you lie and listen to this and goes inwards to understand all the ways in which worries, self-doubt, and negative beliefs about yourself have taken away successes from you...

Longer Pause

And, with this, you know that when you were born, you were free, you were pure, you were joyful, and you had no negative beliefs about yourself. You could say whatever you wanted to say without any apprehensions and inhibitions.

But as you grew up, you learnt the feelings that do not serve any purpose. And because you learnt those while growing up, you can also unlearn those unhelpful thinking patterns and feelings today.

That's right.

Pause

You are naturally a confident person and are capable of doing anything...just like a child. Children are brave and they fear less. Children when born have no self-doubt and they are still capable to seek attention of their parents by smiling, giggling, laughing, and crying. They are confident even when their limbs are small. They cry when hungry and the food comes to them. So easy for them...isn't it?

Pause

Similarly, your natural state is to be confident and brave. You were confident when you were born and you were able to overcome all your doubts, if any and when you were at the age of 3, you could learn new words. Every day, you could express yourself through painting and coloring. You developed motor skills and you learnt to talk, walk, dance, and move your body more. All of that you did with immense natural confidence.

You could not have succeeded if you did not have the confidence and with all the courage to face fears, you could achieve what you needed to achieve.

You were born confident, courageous, and persistent.

Does that mean now it is not there? The part of you having these positive qualities?

Pause

Certainly not, the part is there. It is still there. You just need to find the confident, persistent and courageous part of you.

And, you are now going to look within you…and find that part of you…perhaps it is residing in a small place in your heart or mind.

Longer Pause

Look for it…

Pause

You have found the part somewhere in your body, it is residing in a small room like place. The room is painted pink and red…

And, you go to the room and meet that confident part of you. The part that was born brave and fearless…and persistence was its value.

Pause

You greet the part and you tell the part that how much you have missed it all these years and today, you are going to become one with each other.

The confident part of you agrees to it but before that, it makes a request…a request to drop all the baggage full of self-doubt.

You agree and allow yourself to let go of all the baggage that you have been carrying for so long. It has been so many years that you have it on your shoulders as a backpack.

The backpack has self-doubt, negative beliefs about yourself, and the labels that others have given you about your body and how you look.

Pause

The backpack is full of this and you open it to empty it. You open the main zipper and look for emotional baggage in the side pockets. There are two more pockets inside the big compartment of the bag.

You find many things and one by one you start to take them out and put a fire to them.

Pause

You may find things like "I am not good enough" or "not smart enough" or I am fat, or I am unattractive"

You take all of them out NOW.

Longer Pause

In a moment, you notice that the backpack is all empty and you put the fire to it as well.

Pause

You are free, feeling light and so much more relaxed… and everything seems so much better…and you know from within that you are pure like a child of god or whoever you believe in…

You know you are enough and smart enough and attractive enough because you now go down the memory lane and find so many instances where you believed that you were good enough and smart enough and attractive enough…

Longer Pause

So, the truth is you are good enough, you are smart enough, you are attractive.

This is your new truth…you are brave, confident, smart, attractive, and good enough…

And when you say that the other part of you who sits in a red and pink room, comes running to you…

And you hold that part of you in your arms and give it a tight hug…

Together, you are brave, smart, good enough, attractive and can achieve any goal. On you weight loss journey, with each other's help and support, you can achieve the target of being at your ideal goal so much more easily and faster.

That's right…

In a moment, you will notice both of you becoming one with each other, integrating into one another as one whole complete confident, brave, and joyful individual.

Longer Pause

With every passing day, these positive suggestions are going to go deeper and deeper into your subconscious mind…for your highest good…

Reprogram Your Mind for Long Term Health

And as you continue to relax even more with every breath you take, your each and every breath allows your inner mind to open to absorb all the positive and advantageous ideas and suggestions.

Every heart-beat of yours allows your mind to reinforce these positive suggestions and they get embossed on your mind as permanent ideas... that's right.

These ideas will start to work for your highest good, in the area of your health, body, and weight loss...

And, because your subconscious mind is very powerful, it works in the background as I continue to say the positive words to you for you to lose weight faster...much faster...

You continue to relax more deeply and imagine a beautiful cottage, somewhere...just imagine it with your mind's eye...the eye that takes care of the imagination and helps you daydream...

Imagine the cottage and notice its wall colors from outdoors and perhaps the color of the door and the material it is made of...

Pause

You push open the door and enter the cottage and find yourself in a room with walls, painted with your favorite colors.

One of the walls has large window through which you can see the beautiful lush green garden outside...and on the other wall, you notice a big mirror, which looks exquisite and luxurious...

When you look at the mirror and its beautiful wooden Victorian frame...

On the third wall, is a big control panel...with network switches, wires, many buttons and lights flashing in green and red...

Pause

And ofcourse the other wall has the door from which you entered the cottage...

You look at yourself in the full-length Victorian mirror and notice that you have a body that lets you enjoy everything in the physical world. With this body and limbs, you can walk, run, eat, hold, hug, and do so many other things...

Isn't that wonderful?

Pause

Are you grateful to god for giving you this body to experience life in a better way...Perhaps it weighs more than what it needs to be, but that does not mean, you would not like it...your body gives you so many opportunities to experience things...

Your body is a beautiful creation of god, and you appreciate it even more from today on...and only when you accept something, you can truly work on it to make it better...similarly, today is the day to accept your body just as is and only when you accept it, you will be able to make changes to it..

When you eat proper and exercise, you will be able to reach your ideal goal weight and make your body even better, even more attractive...that's right...

From a beautiful and amazing body, you will be moving to an even better, attractive, slimmer, and fitter body...the body will be healthier and stronger...

The more you appreciate your body now, the more you will be focused to improve it...

Pause

And, in a moment, just so you get motivated to achieve the fitter and attractive body, you can magically see yourself as slimmer, fitter, and healthier at your ideal goal weight as I count from 3 to 1...

3...

2...

And 1...see yourself as fitter and healthier...

Look at your arms, your stomach, your thighs...and your face...

Longer Pause

And as you look at it...you have the power to magically get into the mirror and step in the body of your future self...

Do that now...

Pause

And as you do that, I wonder if you can feel the body of the slimmer self...touch the arms, stomach, thighs, and face...And you can also feel what the slimmer self is feeling...

Light, confident, and attractive...isn't it...

Pause

And you now step out of the mirror and come back to the room...and as you have experienced what it is to be at the ideal goal weight and slimmer, you let your inner mind know all the benefits of being at the goal weight...

Instruct your inner mind to do whatever it takes to give you all the motivation, power, and wisdom to make right food choices, motivate to exercise, and power to take control of life...and eating habits...

Pause

Show your inner mind, the ideal image in the mirror so that it also know what is the goal and what actions are to be taken to achieve that goal...

Your inner mind now knows that this is the ideal image and your inner mind is going to show you all the ways to achieve this ideal self in few months from now…

Pause

Your inner mind helps you change the way you think about food…it helps you change the way food tastes, it helps you make right choices in food, it helps you stay motivated to exercise, it helps you reduce the sugar cravings…

Your inner mind helps you do everything that is important for you to change you look at food and your relationship with it…

And, to help your inner mind do what it needs to do so that you both are in sync with each other to achieve the common goal of losing weight and achieving the ideal goal weight…

You move to the wall with the control panel…

Pause

The control panel has side bars, buttons, flickering lights, and many other things that have different functions…

You know from within that there is a side bar set to a high level…which is a hunger side bar…perhaps on a scale of 1 to 10…it is set at 10.

Bring it down to a level of 5, so that you are hungry only when you are physically hungry and need food to keep going…

Pause

You notice there is a light flickering and flickering of light here only means that you are eating emotionally…or you relate emotions like sadness, loneliness, anger, and similar emotions to eating…fix the light so that it stops flickering…

Pause

You also notice that there is another side bar…that is set at 2 or 3…and that is for exercise.

Bring it up to 8 or 9…so that the motivation to exercise increases. And, you start to exercise daily for at least 30 minutes…

You also notice that there something is jammed up…and that is the metabolism. You need to unblock it so that the metabolism rises up and you start to lose weight faster…

If there is any other fixation your control panel requires, simply fix all of it…

Longer Pause

And, then there is a lock to lock the entire control panel… and you lock it with a big lock…with everything working fine inside of it..

You have now set your body where your metabolism is going to be faster, you will be motivated to exercise, you will make right food choices, you will move your body more, you will sleep on time and feel better after waking up and be absolutely motivated to live your life to the fullest..

Now, back to your room and in front of the mirror…and I wonder if you can look again at yourself in the mirror…

And, now become one with that image of yours…where you are your healthiest, looking absolutely stunning, and attractive.

You love and appreciate your body even more…the inner mind is working harmoniously with your conscious mind to help you meet the common goal of being at the ideal goal weight…

Pause

That's right…

Now, relax even more…as you take each breath…just appreciating your body as it is becoming slimmer and healthier, and attractive…

You know that there is always enough food for you, and plenty of it…and you do not need to overeat to store it as fuel…because there is always enough food for you…

Because, if you accumulate food in your stomach, it turns into fat, and you see it on your body as heavy legs, big stomach, big chest, big face…and with all that do you think you can be the ideal self that you just saw in the mirror?

Longer Pause

With exercise and eating right, you can melt your fat away easily…through excretion…and perhaps you can imagine melting your fat away…like the wax melting off the burning candles…

Pause

And when the fat melts away, you feel amazingly lighter and better…able to move your body faster, exercise better, getting into the clothes easily…And the more you move, the better is the metabolic rate…

With lighter body, you are able to exercise for longer hours and the fat further melts away easily…

From today on, you are going to change your whole body and the feelings of total well being…

You eat healthy, make right food choices, and drink plenty of liquids to always feel lean, attractive and healthy.

Pause

You love yourself and appreciate yourself immensely and with every passing day, this love grows stronger and stronger…

You lose weight steadily every week and you become slimmer and get into the shape that you desire…the extra weight is melting off you…which makes you feel so much better and lighter…

You are in complete control of your eating habits…and you picture yourself becoming attractive and healthy.

Every time in future you want to deviate from your goals, you simply close your eyes and see your ideal self in the vintage mirror. And every time you visit this mirror and see yourself in it, your inner mind magnifies all the benefits of being at the goal weight…

Pause

Now, allow these powerful ideas and suggestions to stay inside a safe place of your mind where they become your new truths…and inhaling and exhaling while you listen to the sound of my voice only means you believe in these ideas and you are going to execute them consciously from today on…

And, every breath allows your mind to strengthen and reinforce these new thoughts, behaviors, and feelings over and over again making them real for you…

That's right..

Letting Go of the Weight Protection

And you continue to take usual breaths and calm your senses..., let's discuss the complexity of your mind.

It is divided into two parts, conscious, and subconscious/unconscious mind. They both have different functions but they both compliment each other. Your conscious mind rationalizes your questions and curiosities whilst solving your problems. In hindsight, your subconscious mind is at work continuously, as it facilitates your regular bodily functions like breathing, blinking, and storing memories.

Pause

At times, your mind can act wild. It consciously desires to achieve success but you find it difficult because your subconscious mind has a different agenda than your conscious mind.

And in such situations...no matter what your subconscious mind is doing, it is doing it with a positive intention even if it feels unsettling or rebellious against your conscious mind. Knowingly, or unknowingly your subconscious mind is always trying to protect you from negativity.

Pause

Let's say that it isn't easy to make your subconscious mind work in a positive way and sync with your conscious mind. However, it can be programmed to work with your conscious mind to give you the best possible results, and you can achieve success in any field you want...especially the area of health, and the area of weight loss.

Pause

The trick to making yourself peaceful is to make changes in a way where you don't offend your subconscious mind. A conscious mind is always curious; it is addicted to figuring out the how's, whys and, what's of everything, especially about the things that bother us. The funny thing about human psychology is that we are more curious about the moon than we are about our inner selves.

Pause

Here's what you should know about your inner conflict - your conscious mind being its curious self will always try to find the root cause of the problem, whilst your subconscious mind may try to prevent it, because you subconsciously know that it might cause more harm than good.

Change is inevitable, but at present, accept that you may not get answers for everything. The old you might have had a different experience with the same problem whereas the new you can solve it quickly.

You can only find peace within yourself when you accept the reason why you don't know certain things. The unknown is what is keeping you happy, sound, and safe. Your happiness should only depend on what is happening at present rather than some past incidents and memories.

Now, I will speak to you about things that you will have a deep understanding of, consciously and subconsciously. Take a sneak peek at your inner self and turn yourself calm and relaxed.

I want you to be aware of your inner self that maintains your eating habits and keeps a check on your weight. You might be imagining it to be a feeling, picture, color, sound, or perhaps even an affirmation. Relax and say to yourself, "I'm conscious about the part of my mind that maintains my eating habits and keeps a check on my weight"

Pause

You need to affirm your consciousness that you are happy to be communicating with it, ask your mind to give you a signal if it feels the same way.

Ask your mind to give you a signal if it is aware of any sensitivity, tension, sensation, colors, pictures that it is in control of your eating habits and weight-loss.

Longer Pause

Thank this part of your mind for everything it has done to protect you in the past. Explain to it now that it is important to make some positive changes to achieve what you want and that you are aware of it in your conscious mind.

Ask your subconscious mind, "Are you willing to try a new strategy where you protect me from negative effects on my weight loss?", it is not easy to communicate with your mind, so ask your subconscious mind to signal you if it is a positive answer.

Pause

Now that you have received a positive answer, ask your mind to make the necessary changes, and to adapt itself to the new strategy. On the other hand, if you didn't receive any signal, then it means that the subconscious mind did not find a strategy that it can adapt to. If the latter one is the case, then go deeper into your subconscious mind, and ask which part of the strategy is the problem, then try altering it.

If it refuses to answer you then ask the creative part of your subconscious mind to create a new strategy. After finding the negotiable strategy, ask your subconscious mind if it would protect you from the negative effects on your weight and if it would allow you to lose weight easily to maintain your target weight. Ask now.

Longer Pause

Ask your subconscious mind if it agrees with the strategies that the creative part came up with. Ask if it is willing to adapt itself to these strategies. If your subconscious mind gives you a green signal, then check within yourself if all aspects of it are acceptable and if they are using the creative part to create new ones.

If they don't agree, then accept what it says about when the strategies will begin to change.

Pause

If you feel the need to seek more strategies, then you are free to do so as I speak. You can either continue to make those subconscious changes or you can rest as I speak. The only thing that can hold you back is if you are subconsciously making all these changes but you are not aware of it consciously.

Weight loss is not something that you can achieve overnight, it takes time and consistency. It will work only if you appreciate the credibility and hard work you are putting into achieving it. In a few weeks when the difference starts to show, you would have convinced yourself that it's all a lie because it is easier and more comfortable to slip back into those damaging patterns.

Pause

You will realize that your changed sub consciousness will protect you from dieting. You will find that eating healthy natural food while doing your regular activities will feed your energy.

You disassociate yourself from the old you who was comfortable with gaining some extra pounds.

You send some positive things to your future self, you notice that you feel more content, and you will start to feel better. From now on, life only gets better and when you hear that critical inner voice you will stop yourself. By being objective, you find an encouraging and constructive way to deal with your problems.

Pause

You start to speak to yourself in a friendlier way because now you accept all the changes. You start to believe in yourself and you accept that you have made a positive change in your life. You notice that you have made a difference by believing in yourself - lookout for the change that increases the energy, it is now returning to you as I count from 5-1.

Eat in Moderation

Now that you are relaxed, you will realize that your mind and body are light...and you continue to breathe normally and focus on the rise and fall of your chest... As you take deep breaths, your mind and body are getting deeply relaxed and lighter...like never before.

Being a foodie, and loving what you eat is a good thing, whereas not knowing when to stop eating can have some serious repercussions on your body. Isn't it?

Pause

Our bodies naturally have reflexes to indicate when you are full, so avoid overeating until you "feel" that you are full. Pay close attention to your reflexes and know when to stop.

Our lives are challenging, we are always busy dealing with the new circumstances, and lifestyles which eventually starts to affect our bodies negatively....

Whether its long days at work, juggling between various tasks on a day, driving down to work, travelling to different cities or countries, spending time with family...we just get lost in our day to day routine, that it gets difficult to pay attention to what we eat, how much we eat, and when we eat...

We eat when we go out or when we are at home...

Pause

Over time, we start ignoring the signals and messages that our bodies are giving us to stop eating. We run over the signs, and we force ourselves with a mouthful which gradually leads to stomach expansion. To feed our stomach accordingly we start to eat more, and the process keeps going on a loop. When we eat more and our stomach expands, we want to eat even more to keep the big stomach full...and then it shows up on our body as fat...

We look big because of our big stomachs...and we continue to overeat even when we have eaten enough...perhaps because we are bored, sad, happy, or just like that...

Pause

It's about time that you change that mentality. Use that "stop eating now" signal to have a healthier and appropriate approach towards food. By making these changes, you can eat less and feel full because you don't want to overeat.

Overeating is toxic and it only leads you to have heavy and unsettling feelings. Your mind and body need to feel light and free to be healthy.

Your subconscious mind knows how a healthy body should look or feel like because it has the blueprint of your body. Only you can bring your body to the right shape and strength with the help of your subconscious mind.

Pause

Cancel out all the noises around you and get deeper inside your subconscious mind. Now, start communicating with it, ask your subconscious mind to alert you when your body has received enough, and the right time to stop eating your meal. As you are communicating, you will notice that your subconscious mind has created a positive response to your request.

This is where your role starts, you will realize that the "stop eating" signal that you have ignored for so long will be faint at first, perhaps even unrecognizable above the clatter of other thoughts that have taken greater priority for so long now.

Pause

Take full responsibility of your mind and body, pay close attention to what kind of signals they are passing to you about your eating habits.

When you are eating, be mindful when that "stop eating now" signal occurs. When you hear it or feel it, respect your body's commands thereby following all the instructions and thank your body for its assistance. I

If you feel like passing on the signal, your body will instantly remind you of it in a powerful manner with the help of your subconscious mind. Your subconscious mind tries to help you by reminding you of your commitment to a healthy life, it reminds you of your responsibilities to make it happen.

Longer Pause

Only when you are committed, you will feel happy, light and free. In the longer run, it is important to feel that lightness, for a calmer, and a less burdened mind. This way you have the lighter body you have always desired for, by burning away that excess weight.

Maintaining good health is only possible if you constantly listen to the cues given by your body for hunger or anything else. Know when to stop eating, how much to eat, and at the right time. Remember, if you are full and if you feel like you are overeating, it is okay to stop.

Find Better Foods

As you continue to listen to me and listen to all the positive suggestions, you start imagining doing things in a completely new way. Explore new horizons, it might seem daunting at first, but the unknown is always scary until you discover it. Once you see that there are millions of possibilities, your whole perspective will be different.

You realize that you have subconsciously been an explorer and a finder in your whole life, without caution, and it has often proven to be the best form of exploration.

Do you remember all your firsts? Do you remember the first time you stepped on the beach sand barefoot? The feeling of that sand beneath your feet, warm, and grainy? The sand moving under your feet as you paddle in the cool sea? Maybe you even had your first sweet candy floss after.

Pause

Experiencing the first snow is always special, do you remember touching it or perhaps observing it closely to see if each flake is unique? Staring at the sky, watching the snowfall on you for the first time is always an amazing memory.

Try and remember the first time you saw a rainbow; you didn't know about any hidden meanings or ambiguity. When you first saw the rainbow and wondered if there was a pot of gold at the end of it. The way those colors integrated into each other intrigued you.

Pause

The only thing standing between you and a pleasurable exploration experience is your irrational fear of the change. Always remember, the journey is more important than the destination, so try to explore new things and enjoy the process thoroughly to make it fun and easy.

Consider yourself to be a baby and try to explore things like they do. For example, the way they develop their ability to taste with their tongues first. Think of an orange, think about how as you peel the orange, the waxy skin even the zest is considered edible in sweet marmalade after removing the soft white pith and before separating each segment. Have you ever observed how within each segment there are hundreds of little pods filled with sweet juice?

Pause

If you pay close attention, you will find a star in the center of the apple if you cut it in the right way but just observing the fresh fruits and vegetables might not be the right way for you. Trying something different, perhaps discovering some new aromas, noticing the subtle sweetness, the delicate sourness, or the warm woody undertones might be the right way for you.

Longer Pause

You might find new things to like. You will find yourself being tempted by the fresh fruits and vegetables of which you never expected to be good. You might find telling yourself, "This might be the food that I'll enjoy." In the quest to find the food you might like, you will have a new experience, you might discover refreshingly amazing things that you can enjoy, swallow, and feel satisfied after eating.

Pause

You will have more faith, trust, and confidence in yourself to find the ability to change and grow, as you explore your interest in growing fresh fruit and vegetables of your own.

Watching them grow, nurturing them with good light, food, and water while caring for them with the love and respect you show to your own body might change you as a person.

Eat Less and Enjoy More

And as you continue to go deeper and deeper with every word I say...you imagine yourself floating on a gorgeous magical cloud...

The cloud is floating across the sky and so are you...sitting comfortably on it...and you can feel the Sunshine on your skin as you continue to float with the cloud...going deeper and deeper, feeling warm sunshine all over you and the cool breeze all around you...

Longer Pause

And now that you are open to receive and are open to the suggestions, I am going to be telling you a beautiful story that will make the whole process of weight loss much easier and automatic...

This story will make your weight loss journey much simpler and at the same time exciting...

Because you will be doing every healthy bit to lose weight and get into the shape that you desire.

Pause

The story is about a small child who loves to have chips and the child asks the parents to give them a full pack of potato chips...

The parents thought about the request for a few moments and told the child the whole pack of chips won't be good for you, but you can definitely have 10 chips and not more than that...

Pause

The child thinks about what the parent just said and the child wonders and thinks ...thinks and wonders...

And then he agrees to take the 10 chips and says to the parent that "I am fine with 10 chips" and the parent serves 10 chips to the child on a plate...

The child looks at them and smells and finds the smell quite enticing...

Pause

The child picks one of the chips and strokes it between the finger and thumb ...perhaps it is tangy or salty or cheesy.

The child puts it in his mouth and feels it with the tongue and crunch...there he goes...delicious...

The child instantly smiles at the parent and says the chip is yum and then another chip gets picked up and relished by the child.

Pause

Slowly and slowly, the child finishes off the plate full of chips…

The child enjoyed each chip's aroma, flavors, texture…and the deliciousness…

And because the child enjoyed each bite and flavors, it took the child 15 minutes to eat it…because he enjoyed each mouthful…feeling absolutely content and satisfied with 10 chips…

Longer Pause

With this, you know that there is a similar child inside you who knows how to enjoy each mouthful and when you eat less and enjoy more, you lose weight…

You eat less and focus on the goodness of each bite and mouthful…when you eat this way, you like food even more and nutritious food becomes tastier for you.

Pause

You eat only when you feel the physical hunger and to keep the energy levels optimum, you eat and not eat when you are hungry emotionally or mentally…

You eat foods that are healthy for your body and give you nutrition to keep your body fueled and healthy at the same time.

Pause

With every passing day, this idea of eating less and enjoying more is getting strengthened and every day for the rest of your healthy life, you eat less and enjoy much more…with every bite and every mouthful…

Pause

You have taken charge of your eating habits and are in complete control of your food intake. You eat small bites to relish the flavors and once you have finished eating to fuel the body, the desire to eat more simply goes away.

And these powerful ideas are going to stick to you and inside of you where this will become your new truth…

I am going to count down from 5 down to 0….these suggestions will go twice as deep into your subconscious mind…

5…going deeper and deeper

4…you eat less and enjoy more…

3…going further deep

2…you chew your food many times and enjoy flavors

1…drifting down…

0…you eat less from today on.

That's right.

Do Not Overeat Junk Food

And as you continue to listen to me, you have realized that it's good to eliminate the cravings of junk food and simply get rid of the rut that you have been having. And perhaps that is all because of your emotions.

Most of the times, eating junk food is related to emotions. When we are sad, we want to eat junk and when we are happy, we again want to celebrate and order in.

Pause

Eating junk when sad distracts us from the negative emotions and when we are done eating the junk food, the emotions of guilt come back and it becomes a vicious cycle.

And now you know that eating junk food does not help, it is all very temporary. No fries, burgers, chips, candies, chocolates can ever make you feel better permanently. In fact, they do more harm than good. Isn't it?

Pause

And you must know that all your feelings come for a reason and they all are good, as they help you guide and then you can take the right actions and take care of yourself.

When you feel sad, you need to introspect why you feel sad and deal with that emotion by taking an action that will make you feel good or better.

Pause

You can change your emotions by changing your thoughts or actions. Perhaps the easier is to take an action and you would feel better.

If you are feeling sad and do not feel like getting out of the bed, do the opposite, get out of the bed no matter what and get on with the day. With this, you will have thoughts about the routine, about taking shower, about working, about everything else but the thought that made you sad.

Pause

This is taking charge of your mind, emotions, and body. You are in control and you know how to control your actions and thoughts for the purpose of the highest good.

Eating does not satisfy any of the negative feelings like sadness, anger, frustration and more…

Eating satisfies your hunger that fuels your body to keep it running.

Eating when used to satisfy emotions make you feel even more negative about yourself. And you do not want to be a part of this cycle. Right?

Pause

You are now ready to start your life that is much more fulfilling and you now know what you have been doing in the past that made you gain weight. One of the ways you can lose weight faster is to completely eliminate junk food.

You are much more capable to change thoughts and actions. When you change your action or thought, you change your feeling.

Pause

Every time you get a thought to order in or have junk food, you distract yourself by doing something that is productive and adds value to your life. It could be watching something funny, speaking to friends or family, singing, listening to music, doing dishes, taking a shower, and many more such activities.

You choose the right actions to distract yourself from the thoughts about having junk food.

You are capable of living your life beautifully and healthily.

With this, you are free from the frustrating cycle of eating junk, feeling happy for a few moments and feeling guilty for a long time.

And as you look at yourself in the mirror, you get into the negative self-talk- why did I eat so much, I am stupid that I ordered so much of food.

Is there a point in such negative self-talk?

Pause

There are so many after-effects of eating junk and the only way to not experience those after-effects is to not have junk food in the first place.

From today on

You are in control

You are in control of your thoughts and emotions

You love yourself a lot more than any junk food

You come first before any food

Change your Eating Habits

As you continue to drift further into a relaxing mood while listening to this recording, with every breath you take your inner mind becomes more open to positivity and new suggestions.

Each pulse of your heart starts encouraging your subconscious to enhance your inner experience and apply the positive affirmations and suggestions to your life.

Pause

These suggestions are not only for now but will be permanently ingrained in your subconscious mind.

The more you will make use of this and concentrate on weight reduction recording, the more deeper the suggestions go into your mind and will work faster for you.

And now you are fascinated about this new positive and constructive approach to reduce weight to acquire the, slim, radiant, and healthy body you always wanted to have.

Pause

So, this is the beginning of a fresh way of thinking, and no doubt you are mesmerized by the effectiveness of the suggestions and most importantly your effort to adapt it in your life that is giving you a new feeling and a new way to live life.

In this process, you are growing into a more successful person that you have always desired to be.

Your goal is much clearer now, to have the perfect shape, health, attractiveness, and most important to lose weight. Losing weight is not your main concern but it's to gain healthy habits, stamina, and endurance. To get fitter and look slimmer and healthier.

Pause

If you continue thinking about losing weight, it might stress you out as the body will offer resistance to your weight loss thoughts. Remember that you are not losing anything but gaining wholesome of healthy things. You are reclaiming control of your life.

Pause

You are a completely changed person and have a new attitude towards your eating habits...

Enjoying food, eating a balanced diet is your habit now and you just love the feeling that you eat only that much amount what your body needs.

You are reflecting on a positive change in terms of what you are eating. It is the same as the situation of the car when your car needs fuel, you provide that and the same rule goes for your body, you eat properly when your body feels hungry. You love eating but only want to have food when your body needs fuel.

Pause

Usually, dieting makes you kill your appetite, and at present, the hunger and appetite, the body's need for food are in coordination.

In your old days, you didn't listen to your desire, you gave more attention to hunger. Hunger is a strong desire or a craving that tempts you to eat more food. Previously you felt hungry not because your body needed fuel perhaps it was because you were bored or you had nothing to do so you decided to eat. These are nothing but Fool's hunger which is the same as Fool's gold.

Pause

Fools gold is something that looks precious but in reality, it has no value. So by this, you should understand that whenever you eat because of emotional causes, or just because it's time to have a meal you are experiencing fools hunger, which is purposeless.

Pause

It's not your fault many of us think that food can fix your aloneness, hesitancy, stress, or boredom but in reality, it is a misconception.

Food only acts as a Fuel for your body and nothing else. Due to this reason, the mind starts to put together the body's psychological need to eat with the physiological need for food. And now as you know the difference among these two, one can never be fooled by fools' hunger.

From now on, you should feel hungry only when the body requires some fuel and it should satisfy the body's temptation with only an appropriate amount of food as per body need.

Pause

You are no longer going to be a fool because of the fool's hunger. You are a spectacular, energetic, distinctive human being with such a conventional routine and your desire to eat is always in the balanced form with your body's need for fuel. So next time when someone asks you for the first time.

Pause

'Are you hungry? You will be chuffed to say NO and from the second time onwards, your stomach will feel full and you will be hungry only when your body needs fuel.

Modifying new interesting eating habits is your new personal goal. This includes habits such as you prepare food at a particular time when you can give complete focus to food, you never eat while standing. There should be no disturbance like watching television, listening to music while one is having their meal. Your focus should be only on the food.

Considerably, you eat only when you are hungry, and not because anyone is asking you to eat .Sometimes when you feel emotionally down, then also you prefer eating. You respect your body now by giving it fuel only when it needs it. The more you have respect for your body, the happier you feel.

Longer Pause

At this point, you eat more heartily than ever before. For the second part of the appetite, you should relish your food and be confident to say "I'm healthy enough to eat properly". Eating food is not just a necessity but you enjoy the food significantly more than before by an impressive new eating habit. Let's take an example you are having a flavorful sandwich, as you take the first bite you put your utensil apart and then you start focusing on how tasty the food is. You concentrate on only that part of food that is inside your mouth.

Pause

As you have developed such great eating habits that now you are chewing food profoundly twice as before. The first bite gives you a feeling of happiness and you extract the strength from the meal. You sense each grain of food, it provokes your smelling sense, and it's nothing but just your first bite. You extract every pleasurable savor that the first bite offers.

Longer Pause

After this only you decide to have another enjoyable bite. As you practice this habit of giving thought to your food, the second part of appetite brings up and lets your brain know that your body is fully fueled, and it's time to stop having another bite.

Pause

This gives you a phenomenal feeling that you are eating less, healthy food, and not to forget appreciating your food countless times with this simple and effective habit.

You have a great understanding of your appetite and can munch whatever and whenever you want. Your mind is your asset and is changing according to your demands and it wants only those foods, which are necessary for your objective of a slim and healthy body.

Pause

Your subconscious only shows interest in foods that are beneficial for your health and not towards unhealthy food. This habit persists throughout your life and you can eat anything you want without stress, as your mind guides you towards healthy eating habits.

Pause

Demerits of dieting are that it will provoke the old theories of your mind which will deprive you of having food and block your improvement. Your bonding with appetite is perfect because of which you eat only when your body demands.

The mind plays a crucial role in judging the relevant food and quantity essential as per your requirement to gain classic shape, size, and weight.

Pause

Your mind is so well trained that it can easily judge that it is self-disciplined, not deprived. Your mind modifies according to the specification; it can deprive you of nothing.

For instance, let us take a situation in which you want to have chocolates as it gives you joy, reduces heart disease risk, provides antioxidants but when consumed in an adequate amount.

If taken more it increases calories, affects teeth however your mind is skilled to conclude the correct amount of chocolate for your health.

Longer Pause

Your thinking process is not the same anymore. Now you no longer feel that you are depriving your body of anything at all besides you feel that you are procuring healthy habits.

You are perplexed by the new trait which is so helpful in gaining the desire that is the perfect shape of your body, ideal size, ideal weight. And it is proceeding so smoothly that it's not even bothering you now. Your subconsciousness is now guiding you to achieve your goals of reducing weight and to develop this weight reduction project.

Pause

Your mind is accordingly restricting the unhealthy idea of dieting. Primarily it is of utmost importance to progress the habit of your eating only at that time when your body needs it. Your inner mind is intensely analyzing your hunger and the body's fuel demand. It is inclined towards the beneficial side of the diet.

Longer Pause

One thing to notice is that few people eat more amount of food and still they are lean and healthy naturally. They never opt for dieting because their eating habit will not affect them. According to slim people, they eat whatever they desire and end up not gaining even an ounce of weight.

Pause

Picture yourself as the person with a lean and attractive body.

Let's do a task, stand in front of the mirror and watch yourself. While you watch yourself, say the same thing as above. Say again and again that you give your body what it needs but still manage not to gain even a single ounce of weight.

Say again

I give my body what it needs but I still manage not to gain even a single ounce of weight.

One more time

I give my body what it needs but still manage not to gain even a single ounce of weight.

Your confidence level is much higher now, as you can eat all you want without worrying about your weight. When you start looking at yourself with such poise and spirit you soon become the one, healthy attractive person.

Pause

As human beings, it is our nature to get attracted or crave for unhealthy food which our body doesn't need. And you ignore such cravings and say NO to stick to the plan of becoming slimmer.

Every single time you use this weight reduction recording or whenever you ease down your whole body and mind are filled with the zeal of these positive suggestions. You get more powerful day by day. Your body starts losing weight much faster than before but in a healthy way.

Pause

When you look at yourself, you find a new version of yourself. You are much slimmer, attractive and it is making you feel stronger, happier, and amazing.

With every breath, you breathe your inner mind and adapt to maximize the effect of this recording in your mind and permanently engrave it in your mind. It's high time you have been practicing this and presently it's just the mind that is automatically working for you.

It's time to cherish and appreciate all you have done and succeeded. And now go back to the real world carrying all new persuasive thought, feeling, and positive force along with you.

Ego Strengthening Script

You are in complete control of your body, it is now relaxed, and you are in a serene state of mind. All your body parts are at ease, and you are at peace, breathing slowly. You start to melt away into a beautiful state of relaxation as you listen to the sound of my voice.

You are drifting further away into a more tranquil state, as you continue to listen to my voice. You are unwinding all the negative and stressful thoughts, and you feel wonderful from inside.

Pause

You are here because you want to feel the positivity in the air around you. You want to feel energetic and zealous to create an optimistic approach to your life. Every word you listen to will leave a long-lasting positive impression on you and your life. You are still here with an open mind because you are open to change.

Pause

Now, you have to do something for yourself, will you? Imagine the person you were two months ago and compare how you as a person have been growing, and how it has improved your life. New day, new you, and you are looking forward to something better every day.

Pause

Take a look at yourself, analyse how your thinking has changed. There is a complete shift in the way your thoughts articulate. You have changed the way you treat others and how you behave with them. You empathize with them now. These changes don't need an extra effort, they are automatic and have been happening unconsciously since your birth. If you look back, you will realize that you are not the same person now as you were as a teenager. Now that you know that change is natural, you think you can change, don't you?

You are in control of your life and you can make some beautiful transformations to any part of your life, can't you?

Pause

Believe that from today, the power to control your life. With this power, you can see beyond the problems and hardships, you will be quick to recognize and tackle them. Try spending time understanding the root of your problems and how to suspend them. Your power gives you the right to choose what the most important and lasting thing is, doesn't it?

With that decision, you take control of your thoughts and life. You decide to focus only on positive things and eliminate the negative thoughts...which give you the ultimate power of not getting influenced, isn't it?

Pause

It feels good to know that no one other than you can influence your feelings, appearance, or what you say unless you let them enter your thought and give them permission, right? This implies that only you have the power to choose how and what affects you.

You are what it takes, you have all the power in the world to take control of your feelings.

Pause

You are a person who easily lets it go and doesn't live in the past because they hold no value in your life. You are strong enough to overcome what the past had to offer you, aren't you?

Even a small change that you make today is going to have a positive impact on your wellbeing and life. As these improvements take place, you get more comfortable and confident about living your life unapologetically.

Your mind has indeed made some transitions and will continue to do so today and in the future as well. You opt to remain upbeat and comfortable. You have signed up for optimism but also energy. You decide to remain outgoing, pleasant, and articulate. You can, can't you?

You are becoming more aware of your physical and emotional health starting from today. Taking care of your emotions and the body properly is your priority, so you go to bed on time for a good sleep and take yourself out every day for at least 30 minutes to revive yourself by doing exercises, cycling, or meditation. You are in control of where your thoughts wander, and you only focus on the positive thoughts that in some way, help you.

You look after yourself well, hence, you deserve to be happy and hopeful, don't you?

You are vigorous, more cheerful, and optimistic from today.

You are slowly but steadily changing and you are not only deeply connected to your connected to your body. You love it and you respect it.

You are now stronger than yesterday…your mind is more at peace and positively charged to take on each day. You are centered, calm, focused, and composed. You are in sync with your inner-self, and you both believe in each other. You completely love yourself.

Difficult times might come in the future where you will feel like there is a parasite of slump growing inside of your mind and body. All you have to do is to think about a tweezer and tweeze that negative thought before it grows on you. The tweezer will act as a shield made out of your positive thoughts. Whenever you are in a puddle use the tweezer again. Close your eyes and remember your affirmations, they will immediately get rid of that parasite and take you to your happy place.

Confidence is the Key to Achieve Anything

Confidence is the key. When you find out that you are confident enough to be in control of your eating habits, you can control your weight.

Pause

The weight loss journey becomes easy for you. You have to be aware that being in control of yourself gives you control over your life, and that focus and will-power make your life easier as you can achieve whatever you want to.

The first step is to figure out what you want to do, and then how you want to do it, only then will you be able to do it. We are all free, and we all have the freedom of choice, so once you realize that the things you thought you couldn't do in the past are only things that you were not choosing to do your life becomes easier.

Pause

Now that you have complete control over your decisions, you can decide whether or not to do these things because your sense of self-worth and self-respect grows day by day as repercussions of your decisions. You become stronger every day when you take control of your life, as you allow yourself to make a conscious decision of who and what you want to be. You completely recognize that you are a product of your thoughts, actions, and attitude.

Times will come where you will be misjudged by someone, but you have to remember that in those moments, the person misjudging you has an error of judgment. It is simply a mistake, and the mistake is committed as a result of their actions, attitude, tremors, and worries. You are not responsible for what others think about you, and their misjudgment doesn't change who you are. You know your worth, and you don't mind people making mistakes.

Pause

You consciously decide and make a decision, and those decisions will help you lose weight. You realize that your self-worth is increasing with every pound of weight you are losing because you feel that every pound is lost because of your decisions. As a result, you are finding it easy to lose weight at a minimum of 1lb per week. You know your body is extremely efficient, so you know exactly know how you are helping it, and soon enough you will start to lose more than 3, 4, or even 5 lbs per week, keeping at least 1lb at a minimum, per week.

One day at a time, as you slowly but steadily start to lose weight, you realize that you are happy with the way you look. You are beginning to get in the shape you have always wanted to be in. It all starts from inside when you realize that you deserve to look good and slim in all those places where you want to lose weight, you are fully in control of your life, eating habits, and that makes you recognize that you feel good about your life when you are this way.

You are in control of your present and future...full control. You realize that you can easily achieve your target weight and shape. The conscious decisions that you make about your eating habits are going to help you achieve your goal. The difficulties you are facing today, your fight against the urge to fall for your temptations will be worth it. You will be gifted with wellbeing, self-worth, self-respect, and immense energy.

More Weight Loss

As you continue to concentrate on your breathing, you will realize that you are relaxing your mind a little bit more every time you are exhaling, and the noise in your head starts to fade away. You will reach a silent state of mind where you can only listen to my voice, and you want to listen to the suggestion that I'm about to give you.

The most important thing to know is that by taking control of your decisions, you are not only losing weight but also finding a permanent solution. This program is designed to help you lose all your fat comfortably but permanently. You are going to completely rejuvenate yourself, as you will be a new person in an absolutely new shape.

Pause

The new eating habits will detox your body, and you will find yourself being content with these new eating habits. This new routine is going to help you enjoy your life, eating the way nature intends you to, and only when it is needed, for the rest of your life.

Pause

In the past, you were consuming more than your body needed for its strength necessities, so the extra energy is now stored as inert fat. Now, if you want to shed pounds and decrease this inert fat, you can burn it up as you meet everyday necessities for energy. You start to eat only what is necessary, and later when you are slim you will realize how much it has helped you burn your weight.

Pause

You are now only focusing on eating less and having a measured diet for a balanced body accompanied by your daily activities. These restrictions are only for your greater good, they will help you burn that inert fat, and lose weight. Although you will eat less than you used to, it will satisfy you to a great extent. You will burn that fat and turn it into your energy. The key is to build a concrete pattern and follow the pattern like it's a compulsion.

Pause

Fat by its very nature contains enormous amounts of putting away vitality. If you start only to consume a tad bit of it every day, you will start to lose your weight little by little every day. Nature has designed the fat stores to last a long time, so weight loss has to be gradual but consistent. It doesn't matter how long it takes to regain your original proportions, you have to hang in there and believe that it will happen gradually but it will stay permanently.

Pause

You have to consistently rearrange your thoughts and bring them to your control so you can watch what you eat. Your food habits need to change forever, and that is how you will see some visible results. When you burn your excess weight, you rediscover the new you. You come out of your cocoon and realize that you are happy with your new body. Your thoughts, ideas, and body image will change completely.

Pause

Calm your mind down and let all these suggestions sink into the deepest parts of your brain. Visualize an image where there is impeccable food you like, there is plenty of it and it's never-ending. Only for you, the food will always be there, so much so that you will never have to worry about starving.

With this amount of food, you will never have to store the food in your body. You are now content knowing that the food is there and you will only eat it when it is necessary because you are done with the rolls of fat on your body parts.

Pause

From now on, storing fat has become unnecessary for you as it burdens your heart and organs. This fat makes you unhealthy and shortens your life expectancy rate. With plenty of food around you, you will never have to worry about storing food in your body again.

Pause

If you didn't already know, there is a small part of your brain that controls the biochemistry of your body and it keep a tab of how much fat you store in your body. This part of the brain is called the hypothalamic area, and the subconscious part that controls your weight based on the body's chemistry is called the hypothalamus area. That is why hypnosis can influence your subconscious mind to control what you eat and how you maintain your weight.

Pause

Presently while affected by entrancing, I am giving you the suggestion to change your body's science with the goal that you can separate these huge storage piles of fat and forestall the repeat of any new and unneeded storage of fat. The fat that has been putting an additional weight and over-burdened your body's functions. Separate and dispose of the unneeded fat stores and change the fat to vital energy. Likewise, get rid of the fat by disposing of it in the form of excretion.

Pause

Excrete it or urinate but get rid of it. Dispose of it inside and out. It activates promptly and you can see the fat dissolving ceaselessly as you use it and discharge it. The globules of fat storages are leaving your body and are being diverted. The fat is burnt and dismissed.

Pause

Don't let the stored fat go to waste, use it as the energy supply that makes you more vigorous. Eliminate any excess fat by eating far less than you need to please yourself with those extra calories. Don't eat anything to replace these fat stores as nothing or no one can force you to do so. You will never need that stored fat to be replaced with anything else ever again.

Pause

Let the injurious and burdensome fat begone forever. Think of yourself as a ship that is overloaded and needs to get rid of the excess cargo, you will realize that for smooth sailing, you will no longer that excess fat. You will only eat small amounts of food until you have used all of this stored energy, and all those ugly excess fats are long gone. From this moment on, you are going to move more, and be more active, for you to feel better than you have ever felt before. You lose the desire for all of the food because eating a small amount of food has helped you reach the shape you want.

Pause

This helps you to eat sensibly and correctly for the rest of your life.

Pause

Changing your food science will help you change your whole body, your feelings, and it will bring you to a wonderful sense of wellbeing. You have started to eat responsibly, you are getting plenty of exercise, you stay hydrated that always makes you feel healthy, slim, and desirable.

Pause

You are taking one day at a time and are losing weight every day. You are now slim and in your desired shape. The excess weight is melting off of you, it is just melting away and disappearing into thin air. You feel stronger every day now that you are in complete control of your eating habits. You visualize yourself the way you are going to be soon - slim, happy, and healthy.

Pause

Now calm your mind down and take in all these suggestions - your mind, body, and spirit are in complete control - your subconscious mind is connected to your hypothalamus to change your body chemistry. Let it monitor your subconscious mind and influence the hypothalamus highly to make this body change. You be in control of your appetite so the fat will be reduced by excretion and burning of stored energy. Eliminate all that extra harmful fat.

Change is the Key

Change is not always pleasant and we fear of something new, although we are completely aware that there is no room for improvement without a little bit of change so if you are having difficulties in some areas, you must change the old toxic patterns.

It's a new day and I'm here with a new suggestion, let's do something entirely different from the routine, something that may be entirely new for you. You might have done something like this in the past. Today I'm asking to see yourself from other's perspectives. Look at yourself as others might see you or as you might be seen in the past.

Longer Pause

Stay away from yourself to witness an entirely new you. Imagine if you separate yourself in time as well as in physical distance, you can see yourself not only as you are at the moment, but as you were yesterday or even far back in childhood. You see yourself grow and what you are capable of doing.

Pause

This is a safe procedure and it is possible because your subconscious mind calculates time and distance differently from the conscious mind. In your conscious mind, everything you see is very concrete and real, the time progresses in an orderly manner - hours, days, weeks, and years.

Although your subconscious mind works in a very different way, you tend to live in the present, but when you are suddenly stressed, you go back to the past. Your response depends on the stress you underwent a year or five years ago.

In your subconscious mind you have a different visualization about yourself. You are sensitive and you can divert immediately if something provokes or excites you. You get back to that childish or infantile behavior and relive an incident with all the sound, fury, and emotion you had the first time you experienced it. In other words, you are like a balloon that is waiting to explode into the past at all times.

Pause

Imagine the future you, the person you will be five years from now. This is not silly, you can totally predict your future depending on your present attitude, behavior, friends, and the situations you create. Although you cannot see the precise names or time, you can see where the future will take you depending on what you are doing now. Time and place are only relative in your subconscious mind. No matter where you are, your attitude is something that cannot be changed throughout your life.

Pause

Imagine yourself to be temporarily outside of your body as if you are a third person and look at yourself, your surroundings, and physical limitations. It is safe to project yourself outside and beyond your normal physical limitations so you can look at yourself and understand. This projection is entirely under your control. You will find it quite easy to separate your spirit and intellect from your body, so do that to be momentarily free from the limitations of it. From this vantage point, you can see yourself from a perspective of your past self to your present self. You will become aware of the program that you had to adapt to keep your physical body alive in a world that is so threatening. You will be able to understand the family's interactions with you as never before.

Pause

From this detached point of view, you can see the defenses that you had created when you were small. You have now outgrown them just as you have outgrown the need for nursing bottles and diapers.

Longer Pause

Projection experience is common to everyone who dreams of changing themselves. A good example is waking up to an abrupt sound from a deep sleep and being momentarily confused about where you are.

You have had the experience of looking at the three-way mirror in a clothing store and seeing yourself from every angle to get a different perspective. Another way to get a projection of yourself is to look into a mirror that shows your reflection in another mirror. Change the angle slightly, and you can see one mirror reflecting in another whole row of mirrors, almost on to eternity.

Now to this picture, imagine adding photographs of yourself in the same pose, but each at different ages of your life. You line them up so that you see the evolution in these mirrors. Depending on how it is placed, you can see yourself projected either into the past or into the future.

Visualize yourself outside your own body with a clear view of your whole life in perspective, you are in possession of all your wisdom, all the learning, and understanding that you have ever gained. In this position, you're now able to influence your destiny by re-programming and upgrading your attitude and defenses. You change yourself everywhere you needed growth and maturity, now all your reactions may come up to your expectations as you relinquish your past.

Encourage yourself, accept yourself, and approve of what you do. See yourself reinforcing the proper eating patterns. You now eat only when you are hungry, and your appetite is easily satisfied. Picture yourself enjoying a dish immensely but only in quantities, you need to fulfill normal physiological requirements, overcome the temptation to eat anything extra. When you observe yourself, it becomes easier to pass on the unnecessary food or drink that will ruin your pattern. As you accept yourself, observe how your need for validation is disappearing quickly and progressively.

Using self-hypnosis is a powerful tool and it is a safe force for you. Its effectiveness increases as you let yourself be projected beyond the limitations of your body. You are accepting the suggestion that you eat only when you truly need food, and that you are satisfied with basic nutrition. You see yourself being increasingly happy with your eating patterns and showing approval of what you do.

Secrets to Build a Healthy Lifestyle

Your positive approach to become a slim, healthy, and attractive body that you desire is going to fetch you results with some of my suggestions. These changes will be permanent in your life if you don't fall into those toxic patterns.

Pause

They are going to give you a thorough effect on the deepest part of your subconscious mind, so they will make an imprint forever. This will become a permanent part of every cell of your brain and your body.

You are going to be amazed by how effective these suggestions are going to be. They will permanently become a part of your everyday life, giving you a brand new pattern, and a train of thoughts, making you effectively successful person.

Pause

Make use of this brand new method that you have never used before. You have begun the first positive approach for obtaining a healthy and attractive lifestyle.

You have chosen this hypnosis as a positive means to obtain this goal because it is a great aid in permanently changing your emotional reactions to food and eating habits. You will realize that hypnosis is the new positive approach to obtain what you desire.

Pause

You have initiated a positive approach toward food and eating. As you begin, this positive attitude toward food, you should also enjoy the food you eat that will help you create a permanent positive change in your eating habits.

You have proven to yourself that eating what is needed will entirely satisfy you; just like drinking all the water, you need. Instead of trying to kill your appetite, treating it as an enemy, you are going to work within the framework of your inborn normal reflexes. You are going to make your appetite your friend while also paying attention to it. Slim people have appetites but they pay attention to them.

Pause

Attractive people also have appetites and they also watch what they eat. Hypnosis helps you in the process of making your appetite your friend rather than an enemy.

Previously, you've been paying attention only to how you can satisfy yourself every time you eat. You used to eat to quench your hunger, but now, you are making a friend of your appetite. You listen to everything that your friend says because you want to keep them safe. When your friend says "I'm hungry," you feed it, and when the hunger disappears, your friend says, "I'm satisfied," you stop. You stop long before your tummy is full because once you have that sensation, it means that you have grossly overeaten. You should bury the need to feel full again.

You see you haven't been paying attention to your appetite all this while because your eating has been driven by emotions rather than hunger. It is only important to eat when your appetite is hungry, but you've been eating even when you were not hungry. You've been eating out of habit when your body didn't need it. You've been eating to satisfy your cravings.

You didn't pay attention when your friend said, "I'm done. I'm satisfied. Stop eating." Your appetite doesn't need to be killed off, in fact it needs some strong reinforcement. Hypnosis will help you make a friend of your appetite, pay attention to the advice of your new friend, and be in sync with your body sensations. If you eat too much against the advice of your new friend, you'll ruin your normal reflexes, and mess the pattern that you have been trying to reinforce.

Pause

It is important to eat only the necessary food and covert fat stores to energy. Drop all your plans of dieting, otherwise, your old instinct for self-preservation will come into the frame. This plan can spoil all of the positive results that you wish to gain from hypnosis. It is important for you to develop that habit now; that you're always going to eat all that you need. Under hypnosis, you can reinforce the normal feedback mechanisms, the checks, and balances that tell you when you need food.

Hypnosis may be strong, but it cannot overcome the basic instincts for survival, and the strongest instinct is self-preservation. To your surprise, your great concern about being overweight leads to sporadic dieting, and this gradually turns into starvation. Starvation demands defence, it brings out the instinct of self-survival, and this instinct is responsible for maintaining your excess weight.

You must have heard that slim people eat everything they want but they manage to stay healthy and attractive. Now, visualize yourself to be that slim person who is healthy, and attractive that you aspire to be. Pretend that you are a slim person, you will soon become one.

Pause

Overweight is primarily not a dietary problem, but an emotional problem that you must resolve right now to give up dieting forever. You will form a pattern to eat all you need when your body needs it by paying close attention to your appetite, and trusting your reflexes by reinforcing the sensation. Even if the weight loss process is slow initially, you will catch up eventually.

Pause

You will be slim, healthy, and attractive as you will feel wonderful in every way. The very word diet will be removed from your vocabulary as dieting only makes you think of growing hungry and giving up food. It will trigger your anxiety about starvation which brings forth the instinct of self-preservation, so your affirmation should be to be through with dieting; you are through with dieting forever.

Hypnosis will not only feed your hunger but will also keep your pattern in track while giving you a wonderful feeling of wellbeing. Remember, the very word diet is negative as it threatens you with denial of food, and death. Hypnosis is a positive word; it makes you relax, comfortable, and makes you feel alive. Diets fail eventually; hypnosis can be slow but you are headed towards permanent success with it. Diet brings nothing but starvation to the table which leads to overeating and obesity. Hypnosis brings satisfaction and an unsaid calmness which leads to relaxation. It helps you bring positive changes to your body. The age-old urge to diet is completely buried for now, and you realize that the real answer is in restoring normal reflexes. You will concentrate on that by obeying every suggestion I give you, for hypnosis, as it is the only positive approach. Hypnotic suggestions will rapidly bring a change to your lifestyle by instilling a necessary pattern to ensure a permanently slim, healthy, and attractive body that you desire.

Pause

Every time you are tempted to eat or drink anything that you know will have a negative effect on your pattern, you will say "no" and stick by it, because the rewards are much more important to you than feeding your temptations.

The reward of being slender, more desirable, and sexier are more important to you than eating all the food that you know is wrong for you.

The Road of Life

When your objective is clear you don't stop until you get it and that is why you are concentrating on hearing to this recording as you have strong enthusiasm for this prime goal in your life.

Pause

Your goal is to attain and sustain the optimal, perfect, healthy weight for yourself. You may find yourself having a conversation about what you think of your weight problem. The purpose of listening to this recording is to build an optimistic attitude and encourage you to have a perfect, lean, appealing, strong body. You should understand that it is your birthright to have a healthy body and mind.

Pause

Now I want you to take a look at your weight problem as an overload that turned out to be a serious issue that you have been carrying for a long time. The overload can be everything and anything that makes much sense to you like gibber stone, a heavy backpack, a can of worms, or any object that represents the weight problem in your mind. This object signifies not only your weight issues but the various problems you have been facing until now.

Pause

It calls attention to the fact of the matter whether you are cognizant about the issue or not. The relevance of this object is not just limited to this, but it shows concern about all your routine practice that has contributory cause for weight gain, whatever harm, suffering that this excess weight is causing. Overweight not only harms physiologically but also psychologically.

To cut a long story short this object implies all the complications and all its root and consequence. Let your mind imagine yourself and the object which represents this complete weight problem in your mind.

Pause

Let your life force conceptualize an object which represents the outcome of the weight problem and try to work with that object. Try to consider every important point, list down all potential factors that are involved. You may not be able to recognize why this object is indicating your weight issues but your subconscious understands it ideally. First and foremost remember all the difficulties you have been facing, and be conscious about the duration through which you have been carrying this. And always remember the pain you have been through to adapt it in your life.

Pause

Now feature your life as it is a road, long, splendid, winding road...it extends beyond your imagination, a never-ending road. Roads are pretty similar to our life. Ans you are standing at a mark which is labeled as "today". Even now you are carrying your object of the weight problem.

This situation makes you think that life would be much easier and happening if you didn't have this weight problem. You can appreciate your life much better with a beautiful, healthy body.

Looking at the scenario your mind decides that it can no longer accept or deal with weight problems.

Pause

Its been a long time since you have been holding this issue, just release that object with weight issues from your mind and life.

Now keep aside this object on side of the road and let it leave you alone. As you are keeping down the representative of your problem, you are abandoning the entire weight problem permanently. Forget every trouble, complication, effects about it. Just let it go.

Pause

After leaving everything behind, you feel relaxed and satisfied. There is happiness after removing the burden. You are feeling so light and independent that you could flow like a helium balloon.

Presently , you are free from the considerable burden so just cherish this moment and float in the sky go higher and higher. And start looking at the complete road of your life below you from the sky.

Be so enthusiastic that you can't see any problem from your past, just see the road of life outspread there. Keep flying till you have the power to produce deep emotion with your soul. Always remember that road of life is continuous, it can only take you to places such as birth, childhood, old age, death. As you float high in the sky, there is a feeling of progression, you feel as if you are associated with someone who is immensely larger than you. You are looking back about something invaluable...feeling of refined. And you carry on floating in the feeling of being pure, peaceful with every single breath.

Pause

At this moment in time, you are floating steadily beside you notice the road of your life at that point which is marked 'today". And you will notice that the object of the weight problem is not anything but itty-bitty stone underneath you. Its high time to eradicate the trouble from your life lastingly.

Did you notice that you solved the issue with that object in a small distance and a short duration of time on the road of your life? You have eliminated it for all time. I can't mention exactly the time when you will resolve this serious matter of weight problem permanently from your life.

You can travel into your future to the place where you left the object [representative of weight problem] and surprisingly there won't be anything that bothers you. Just keep moving forward in the floating sky till you reach your destination and it will show that the object with a weight problem has just disappeared.

Pause

Travel to a time in the future where you are no longer facing your weight problem. You are doing it by floating above your life path, looking down to find the exact spot where you have finally lost the miserable weight object. It is only a little ahead; the spot where you have lost sight of the weight object and all that it represents.

Pause

As you reach this place, floating high over it, I want you to get to know yourself in this time. Now imagine floating down to reach this place where your weight object and all that it represents is finally gone. Float down to meet this future self who is now wiser, more accomplished you who is now rid of the weight object.

Pause

You are awaited in the future; after all it is your future self. Your visit is expected. Notice the warmth as the future-self welcomes you. You can see pure love and a hundred percent acceptance for yourself, for your entire being. This acceptance comes from a place of knowledge.

Your future self knows that it would've never been possible to exist if it wasn't for you. You had to be exactly how you are now for your future self to exit in such a place. Let this acceptance for yourself and your body flow into you.

Pause

Accept this acceptance for yourself. In this moment, look at yourself and realize that these feelings of acceptance and self-love were always yours. This is how you were meant to feel for every part of yourself.

Look at your future self and take in how much it has changed from now. The person standing strong in the future is a light, slender, healthy looking you. Your future self has an attractive body and earning that body is your goal. Notice how well the clothes fit your future self and how well he/she moves. Fell the air of strength, confidence and self-esteem that surrounds you in the near future and understand that this is how God wanted you to be.

Get a hold of your future self and ask him/her: "How do you feel now that you have finally resolved the weight problem completely?" The answer you will get is that it feels great to be your true self a little ahead in the future. This is the true feeling of being alive to live with your lighter, slender self. Fill up your heart with the optimism and the good feeling of being in the future. Power up your mind instructing it to do whatever it takes in order to bring out this positivity and make your body lighter and wonderful permanently.

Seek help from your future self and ask for clues, hints or instruction that could help you get closer to that future self and your ideal body. Give your future self a moment to go through any mistakes that he/she made getting to this place. Allow yourself to take your own advice and resolve any mistakes regarding food, changing tastes, healing emotions and looking for creative ways to let go of any stress. Let your conscious guide you towards a healthy, natural relationship with food and body; freeing yourself of guilt regarding errors of the past. You are now entering a new phase your life, in a healthy future with a deep, growing appreciation for the miracle that your life is.

You simply continue breathing peacefully if these thoughts are acceptable to your mind. Every breath you take is a step of your mind resolving and dissolving away your weight problems and reinforce every positive thought you are picking up from this recording. Breath by breath you are earning a lighter heart, lighter mind, lighter spirit and body.

Pause

It is now time to return to the outside world. But you need to remember that you can reach out to your future self anytime you want to take in this feeling of self-love and positivity. All it takes is for you to close your eyes in a safe places and visualize yourself coming down the path of your life, where your future self waits for you with arms wide open.

You can do so either by listening to this recording or simply by thinking of the road of your life with your eyes closed. You are magnifying and accelerating your journey to your lighter, slender future self every time you close your eyes. Everything you need is just a few steps away from you.

Low Carb Diet

I would like you to take a moment here to notice how relaxed your body is… Every inch of your being is at peace… allow this peacefulness to sink in completely, in your head, your neck, your shoulders, your chest, your arms, your waist, your legs… all the way to the tips of your toes… you are so relaxed now that it feels as if you floating like a soft white cloud in the clear blue sky… flowing with the breeze… following the sound of my voice… a voice that you trust to guide you on this journey… a voice that will guide you on your path to achieving a healthier, fitter, and more active body.

Your mind is now open and focused on the suggestions I give… accepting them and taking you twice as deep with every word you hear… helping you relax and feel more comfortable… as you drifter further and further, deeper and deeper into this beautiful state of relaxation.

Creative Visualization

And as this wonderful state of relaxation becomes one with you… I wonder if you can imagine yourself standing in front of a mirror covered with a piece of cloth… slowly and steadily I would like you to move closer to the mirror and pull away the cloth covering it… and as soon as you remove the cloth, you shall see the reflection of a new you… with a fitter body, toned arms and legs… taut muscles and a flat tummy… a version of a perfect you… standing right there in front of you in all glory… I would like you to blink your eyes like the shutter of a camera and let this image of you be imprinted forever in your mind… an image that motivates you and makes you happier… that's right.

As you save this image in your mind where it feels comfortable… it is now time to hop onto a joyride… imagine a dining table in front of you full of fresh fruits and veggies… they look so inviting that you move closer to take a better look at them… and as you move along the side of the table you get a closer look at them… fresh, nutritious, and delicious vegetables… fresh, juicy, and scrumptious fruits… straight from the farm to your table… rich in proteins and vitamins, and less on carbs… you can see carrots, broccoli, kale… shining with their vibrant colors…

look closely, listen to them as they whisper to you with joy, "eat me!" You feel tempted to have a taste and pamper your body… that fit and fabulous body you just saved a picture of… so you go ahead and bite into a carrot and as soon as it touches your tongue, you feel its magical taste blowing you away… tempting you to eat more of it… with each bite your taste buds jump with joy… it's a fun riot in your mouth and you are enjoying it more with each passing moment… and as you continue to enjoy this moment, you begin to realize all that you had been missing out on… and with that realization comes a determination to switch to a low-carb diet…

Metaphor

But before you do that I would like you to imagine a tiny version of yourself hopping into a cart loaded with high-carb fatty food making your way through the digestive system of your body… as this food begins its journey through the mouth, into the throat, and down into the stomach, you begin to see how it gets broken down by the various enzymes into large chunks of sugar…

these chunks begin to break down into smaller bits and begin to make their way into your bloodstream... look closely here and you will notice that some of them are good and get absorbed into your body cells giving your cells an energy boost... but you will now notice how the remaining sugar molecules are beginning to remove their masks to reveal villainous and unhealthy molecules that are about to make their way into your liver and muscles to get accumulated as fat... your body is working too hard to digest them... it has to secrete larger than normal quantities of insulin to fight these unhealthy molecules... your body is working much harder than it should... you feel aghast at the sight of this fat that can destroy your body, making you realize the sinful nature of high-carb foods.

But now that you have decided to switch to a low-carb diet... let us take a journey through your digestive system once more... This time, with low-carb food. These foods, when broken down, result in a minuscule amount of sugar molecules... as such, your body needs less effort and less insulin to work on them... this means your body can rest easy and breathe easy... but your body cells still need energy and as such, the fat reserves of your body will be broken down now that your body feels stronger... melting away all the unwanted calories... helping your body breathe easy, feel lighter, fitter, and stronger than ever...

Now that you have seen the life-changing benefits of low-carb diet coupled with staying hydrated with the help of lots of water and fluids... your resolve to switch to it is stronger than ever...

So now, as you stand in front of the mirror once again, imagining yourself wearing that favorite dress of yours... and how it fits perfectly... you realize that eating right is your new motto in life now... and as these words start to sink in you can feel yourself transforming from within... into a cheerful and liberated version of yourself. And each suggestion I have given, has been deeply engraved into your mind... every letter, every word has etched itself in every inch of your being... there is no turning back now... you eat right... you will not let this new, free, vibrant version of you down...

Direct Suggestions

Repeat the following suggestions in your mind three times now...

I am in love with low calorie food, and I feel great all the time.

I am in love with low calorie food, and I feel great all the time.

I am in love with low calorie food, and I feel great all the time.

Awesome work!

You are in love with low calorie food.

You make better food choices because you love every inch of yourself. Inside out!

Reinforcement Script

And, with every breath you take, you continue to go deeper and deeper with every breath you take and with every word I say. You are drifting into a deeper and even more relaxed state of mind. And that only means, you are focused on the goal of achieving your ideal goal weight.

It feels so amazing to feel this way, absolutely relaxed and calm, knowing that you are on the right track to be what you want to be. A person who is in control of their life, knows what to eat and what not to eat, be aware of the signal from the brain when the tummy is full of food and you stop. You listen to the signal...and you stop.

Pause

You sleep 7 to 8 hours every night and you wake up feeling fresh and motivated to achieve your daily weight loss goals. You take right actions, be in control, and eat nutritious food and exercise.

You are reinforcing now what all you have learnt. You have learnt to let go of all the unwanted beliefs and labels that you or people may have given you about your appearance. Anything that made you doubt yourself, you have already released that.

You know the importance of having smaller portions and how it can boost the metabolism and how you easily you can then lose weight.

You can let go of all the tension and your body and mind are in sync. Your mind is listening to me and it gets easier to fall into a beautiful state of relaxation...and be more aware at the same time of all the suggestions.

Pause

So, just let go and go with the flow and think about nothing, nothing at all as all you need to do is to simply relax and let go...

Pause

I congratulate you on your decision to live your life beautifully and in a healthier way. You have made this decision to be at your ideal goal weight that will not only make you look attractive but also make you feel confident, healthier, and smarter.

Your old habits are simply fading away and you are creating better habits for yourself. You know you can unlearn that you learnt which did not do much good to you and instead learn that can do much good to you. With that, you can achieve a body and mind that you always desired.

And, again, let's reinforce your future image in your mind now, enjoying all the successes in future.

Imagine your future image now.

Longer Pause

That's right. Look at yourself and see your body and what you are wearing. Are you walking and talking more confidently? Look what people around you, your friends and family are saying looking at you? Are they appreciating and getting inspired?

Longer Pause

At the ideal goal weight, what do you notice? What are you doing? What activities are you doing? Outdoor and indoor activities, perhaps all the adventures that intrigue you. Are you able to do all of that at your ideal goal weight?

I am sure, you are

Longer Pause

Imagine yourself at the beach. See, what you are wearing? See how great you feel with minimal cloth to soak up the sun. Make that picture of yours really vivid and magnify it.

Pause

And you have achieved all this because you overcame all your old toxic patterns and limiting beliefs, and bad habits. You took charge of your life and see where have you reached? Your ideal body weight! From today on, you look forward to a beautiful future where you notice yourself as a healthy person, enjoying all the good things in life. Feeling absolutely confident and attractive.

Every passing day helps you to get rid of old thinking patters and now imagine that you are on a bridge...and as you see yourself on a bridge that in the front of the bridge is a beautiful garden.

The garden that looks extraordinary in every way...and when you look behind, you notice a place that looks dingy, dull, and lifeless.

You are on the middle of the bridge...awaiting to get to the beautiful garden.

Pause

In a moment, you reach the garden...and look around. It looks beautiful with magic all around you. You see flowers, birds, and trees that look extraordinary in every way. They have colors that you have not seen before. This is a special place...a place full of wonder and magic.

And, here you notice your future self, doing what he had done in the past few months. And you observe your future self closely...and its habits.

Your future-self, eats healthy nutritious food and does not snack between meals. Your future self, drinks 8-10 glasses of water every day to get rid of toxins, which has promoted weight loss.

Your future self sleeps 7-8 hours every night and exercises every day. You notice your future self to be extra ordinarily confident and attractive. Your future self also practices mindfulness.

Learning from your future self, you have decided to practice mindfulness, exercise regularly, sleep well, eat healthy, and be aware of your emotions and thoughts.

Weight Loss Affirmations

1. Your body is getting fitter with every passing day and it makes you feel confident. (7 seconds pause)
2. You are making choices that carry you farther in your weight loss journey. (7 seconds pause)
3. Your weight loss journey has the support of everyone around you. (7 seconds pause)
4. You are consistently envisioning yourself at your ideal weight. (7 seconds pause)
5. You are entirely capable of losing weight in order to attain your ideal weight. (7 seconds pause)
6. You are sufficient on your own. (7 seconds pause)
7. Weight loss comes as easy and natural as breathing air for you. (7 seconds pause)
8. Your standard of life and health is naturally rising with this journey.. (7 seconds pause)
9. The idea of achieving and maintaining your ideal weight with ease makes you feel excited. (7 seconds pause)
10. The weight that is you lose now, you are losing it for good. (7 seconds pause)
11. You love your body the right way. You are helping it through this journey of losing weight. (7 seconds pause)
12. You easily burn fat. (7 seconds pause)
13. You listen and answer your body's needs. (7 seconds pause)
14. You have an earnest drive to move ahead into achieving your weight loss goal. (7 seconds pause)
15. You are committing yourself to a lifestyle that doesn't only bring good health and weight loss but also higher self-confidence and self-esteem. (7 seconds pause)
16. The right proportion of food needed for weight loss is satisfactory for your appetite. (7 seconds pause)
17. Eating healthy and going to the gym are activities that you enjoy. (7 seconds pause)
18. You are helping your body recover well each day as you allow yourself to take sound sleep and relax each day. (7 seconds pause)
19. The content you read and watch are of the nature which provides you knowledge and ideas of effective weight loss. (7 seconds pause)
20. You are greatly inspired by the idea of the long-term positive effects your weight loss that will incur on your body. (7 seconds pause)
21. You are setting a list of realistic yet challenging goals for yourself that inspire you move along this journey. (7 seconds pause)
22. You can never take your eyes off your goal of weight loss. (7 seconds pause)
23. Your weight loss goal is a passionate drive for your heart and soul. (7 seconds pause)
24. You can clearly perceive the positives of this journey that outweigh the negative. (7 seconds pause)
25. This change of lifestyle to lose weight makes you feel grateful. You love losing weight. (7 seconds pause)
26. You feel great to stand witness to the improvement this journey brings to your health and life. (7 seconds pause)
27. You can rely on yourself to only make choices that help you lose weight. (7 seconds pause)

28. You are excited by this journey towards weight loss and love every step you take towards this goal. (7 seconds pause)
29. You have the image of being fit and healthy in your mind and all your thoughts are constantly revolving around this positive image. (7 seconds pause)
30. You find it reinforcing to share your insights and tips with you fellow friends. (7 seconds pause)
31. You are glad to have a body that is able to exercise and lose weight effectively. (7 seconds pause)
32. You are grateful for the numerous means of help you get in forms of tools and tips to help you get fit. (7 seconds pause)
33. All your cells feel healthy and vibrant; and so do you. (7 seconds pause)
34. You are the one that controls your weight. (7 seconds pause)
35. You have efficiently worked you exercise and workout routine into your daily life schedule. (7 seconds pause)
36. It is you that has a command over your body and mind; not the other way around. (7 seconds pause)
37. You are getting closer each day to your ideal goal weight (7 seconds pause)
38. You see every day as an opportunity to begin with positive thoughts and stability in life. (7 seconds pause)
39. You are eating perfectly and proper proportions of food on your own. (7 seconds pause)
40. You hold on to the positive thoughts that give you hope. Your goals are achievable and you are sure of this. (7 seconds pause)
41. You have based your core values around your health and fitness. This helps you naturally make choices towards your weight loss journey. (7 seconds pause)
42. You are developing an appetite for healthy, whole food. (7 seconds pause)
43. Working out comes natural to you. (7 seconds pause)
44. It doesn't bother you to work out and it comes to you with ease. (7 seconds pause)
45. Each day, you become more active physically. (7 seconds pause)
46. Your food is to fuel your body, not a means to suppress your emotions. (7 seconds pause)
47. Your body's metabolism helps you burn fat as it is high. It helps you lose weight faster. (7 seconds pause)
48. Your lifestyle is changing forever. It is a commitment to a healthy lifestyle and not just a diet plan. (7 seconds pause)
49. You can envision fat melting off your body every day. (7 seconds pause)
50. You are making a promise to love yourself as you go ahead in this journey. (7 seconds pause)
51. Your body is going to see positive changes and it is safe to do so. (7 seconds pause)
52. You are losing weight with ease as you are getting help form your well working cardiovascular system. (7 seconds pause)
53. Your priority is to move forward and make progress even if it's not perfect. (7 seconds pause)
54. You understand that everyone is unique. You hold no expectations from your body to be quick; only that it loses weight and that it keeps on happening. (7 seconds pause)
55. You are receiving help from the universe as it conspires to help you lose weight. (7 seconds pause)
56. You are on this journey in which your dedication and commitment to your health is inspiring to others. (7 seconds pause)

57. You enjoy eating healthy food. (7 seconds pause)
58. You are confident that you will be able to transform your body and mind with your abilities. (7 seconds pause)
59. You are inspired and motivated by the goals you set for yourself on this journey of weight loss. (7 seconds pause)
60. You are becoming better each day, gaining control over your weight loss. (7 seconds pause)
61. You are not feeding yourself out of boredom, but because your body needs it. (7 seconds pause)
62. You have set your feelings and emotions affirm around your weight loss. (7 seconds pause)
63. You are moving at a pace which is perfect for your body, not because you are ashamed of your body. (7 seconds pause)
64. You don't feel the need to rush into losing weight. You understand that the right way is losing weight slowly, in a healthy manner. (7 seconds pause)
65. You prefer progress over perfection. (7 seconds pause)
66. Your journey to effective weight loss is guided by the universe. (7 seconds pause)
67. You enjoy watching how your body transforms and your clothes start to fit better. (7 seconds pause)
68. Each day, it becomes easier for you to lose weight. (7 seconds pause)
69. There is a great positive shift in your body and mind that can only be felt. (7 seconds pause)
70. Each day, you get a little closer to your ideal weight. (7 seconds pause)
71. You don't feel the need to finish the entire plate. You only eat what you need for your weight loss. (7 seconds pause)
72. You pre plan your meals for the week to help you create an effective weight loss plan to achieve a healthier body. (7 seconds pause)
73. You no longer feel the need of extra weight around your body in order to protect it. (7 seconds pause)
74. Your strong new self makes you feel protected and safe. (7 seconds pause)
75. Your mental and physical power are all you need for an effective, long lasting weight loss. (7 seconds pause)
76. You can see your fat loss progress each day and it is an amazing feeling! (7 seconds pause)
77. Your mirror is a reflection of a warrior, a champion who is standing there at his/her perfect body weight. (7 seconds pause)
78. Your mind might try and sabotage your efforts, but you can only see your past accomplishments at these moments. (7 seconds pause)
79. You are following only the best health and fitness influencers and coaches online on social media platforms. (7 seconds pause)
80. Your body is amazing and you love it for how it is. (7 seconds pause)
81. You are restoring your body by eating healthy. You are helping it heal. (7 seconds pause)
82. Your first thoughts when you wake up in the morning are of body positivity on your weight loss journey. (7 seconds pause)
83. You will find it easier every day to let go of all your old habits. (7 seconds pause)
84. Your health is consistently improving every day. (7 seconds pause)
85. You are focused only on the positives of losing weight. (7 seconds pause)

86. You have a big reason to start this weight loss journey. It is strong enough to pull you through all the tough times. (7 seconds pause)
87. You have no difficulty refusing to people and food when needed. (7 seconds pause)
88. You are a winner. You don't stop until you've won. (7 seconds pause)
89. You are attracting people who will help you through this journey. (7 seconds pause)
90. Your intuitions are your guiding light through this journey of weight loss and a better, healthier life. (7 seconds pause)
91. You choose to challenge your mind and body with fitness and better health choices. (7 seconds pause)
92. You are making new choices for your health and wellness and your body has started to quickly adapt to these changes. (7 seconds pause)
93. You are sure without a doubt that you will do the right thing and achieve your goals. (7 seconds pause)
94. Your weight loss is not a sprint, but a marathon. You are not going to rush. Your decisions are going to be for your long-term health benefit. (7 seconds pause)
95. Your focus always needs to be the positive aspects of your weight loss journey. (7 seconds pause)
96. You are gifting yourself a strong, sturdy and healthy body and lifestyle. (7 seconds pause)
97. You are thankful that you have health and fitness as such a big part of your life. (7 seconds pause)
98. You are your biggest admirer. (7 seconds pause)
99. Your muscles toning up inspire you. (7 seconds pause)
100. Every ounce of fat that you lose becomes a boost to your motivation. (7 seconds pause)
101. This journey of weight loss is a wake-up call for the giant within you. (7 seconds pause)
102. You move on further towards your next win inspired and encouraged by your progress. (7 seconds pause)
103. You easily find food that is healthy for your body and it helps with your weight loss. (7 seconds pause)
104. You are fine with taking a very small step now as you know that it will later become running strides. (7 seconds pause)
105. Weight loss to you is not a destination to arrive upon, but a journey. (7 seconds pause)
106. Your body detoxifies perfectly, helping you lose weight. (7 seconds pause)
107. Your body is strong and healthy. You admire its way of functioning. (7 seconds pause)
108. It serves you well in the long run to have friends who are going through the same journey as yours. They become your accountability partners. (7 seconds pause)
109. You listen and watch things that are going to reinforce your already powerful mind. It helps you through your weight loss journey. (7 seconds pause)
110. Every win, weather big or small, is going to make difference to your body. (7 seconds pause)
111. You are in awe of the way you have transformed your life with this commitment to lose weight. (7 seconds pause)

112.   Every neurotransmitter in your body is firing you up with energy and making you feel great all day long. (7 seconds pause)

113.   You can feel an amazing transformation taking place in and out of the gym. (7 seconds pause)

114.   Your gym has become an amazing place for you to go, get fit with people who can become supportive positive friends. (7 seconds pause)

115.   You engage in all calorie burning activities with great enthusiasm. (7 seconds pause)

116.   Your weight loss journey let's you laugh in the face of any challenges that you face. (7 seconds pause)

117.   You no more have any limiting beliefs around the matter of weight loss and failure. (7 seconds pause)

118.   You hear encouraging words from your friends about your weight loss. (7 seconds pause)

119.   They don't forget to remind you of how great you look while on this journey. 7 seconds pause)

120.   You resolve any hungers pangs by meditating or hydrating your body. (7 seconds pause)

121.   All your old habits are getting replaced by healthy habits that make your weight loss easier. (7 seconds pause)

122.   You feel that you've been immensely blessed on your weight loss journey. (7 seconds pause)

123.   You coach yourself and keep on motivating yourself on your journey. (7 seconds pause)

124.   Every passing day makes it even easier for you to refuse any unhealthy food. (7 seconds pause)

125.   You are aligning your home with your health and fitness goals. (7 seconds pause)

126.   You have discovered that your passion lies with health and wellness. (7 seconds pause)

127.   You seek inspiration in new ways everyday to push yourself forward on the weight loss journey. (7 seconds pause)

128.   You are surprised by your will to go to the gym. (7 seconds pause)

129.   The dreaded thought of weight loss and fitness has now become lighter and easier for you to explore. (7 seconds pause)

130.   You rule your own fate and soul. (7 seconds pause)

131.   You now have people who hold you accountable for your goals. (7 seconds pause)

132.   You are now unstoppable on this journey. (7 seconds pause)

133.   You are now letting the world in as you would let it with your perfect weight. (7 seconds pause)

134.   As you see your body slimming down, you look and feel stunning. (7 seconds pause)

135.   You have stopped engaging in any negative self-talk and all you see in yourself is a champion. (7 seconds pause)

136.   Your reflection looks like a thinner self to you. (7 seconds pause)

137.   You are striving hard towards your fat reduction goal, supported by perfectly synced body and mind. (7 seconds pause)

138.   Your entire focus is on how well your clothes fit you and not on what the scale tells you. (7 seconds pause)

139.   You are powerful and confident in your body. (7 seconds pause)

140.   Your mornings are cheerful with exciting possibilities that the day holds for you. (7 seconds pause)

141.   You love how your body is slim, slender and toned like that of an athlete. (7 seconds pause)

142.   You receive words of encouragement from strangers and friends about your weight loss and fitness. (7 seconds pause)

143.   Even a small step forward is a step closer to success. Any progress is good progress. (7 seconds pause)

144.   You are limitless. Nothing can stop you from achieving what you want. (7 seconds pause)

145.   The clothes you love fit you a lot better now as you are losing weight. (7 seconds pause)

146.   You are in good health and wellness and that is how it will always be. (7 seconds pause)

147.   Your need for long term sustainable results cannot be fulfilled by fad diets or gimmicks. They are becoming meaning less to you. (7 seconds pause)

148.   Your eyes are open to everything positive that weight loss has brought into your life. (7 seconds pause)

149.   The journey that you are taking is for yourself, for the betterment of your mind and body. (7 seconds pause)

150.   You are shedding away all the guilt and negativity that surrounds food right away. (7 seconds pause)

151.   The new clothes that you have bought for yourself make you look amazing! You are glad the old ones don't fit you anymore. (7 seconds pause)

152.   You are breathing in wellness and exhaling fat. (7 seconds pause)

153.   You feel great as you intake food that nourishes your body and helps you lose fat. (7 seconds pause)

154.   You are becoming the best version of yourself and it is a thrilling feeling. (7 seconds pause)

155.   You have gained momentum and changed things to be more positive in this weight loss journey. (7 seconds pause)

156.   Chewing your food completely makes you feel full with less food. (7 seconds pause)

157.   Your perfect working digestive track aids you in fast and effective weight loss. (7 seconds pause)

158.   You have lost the taste you had for unhealthy food. (7 seconds pause)

159.   The realization that unhealthy food makes you feel bad about yourself has helped you let go of bad food habits. (7 seconds pause)

160.   Your body is a temple in which your soul resides in good health. You have massive gratitude and respect for it. (7 seconds pause)

161.   You are in awe of the long way that you have come in this weight loss journey. (7 seconds pause)

162.   You feel that God is constantly holding onto you through this journey, giving you support. (7 seconds pause)

163. You will achieve perfect health and wellness with you power to do so. You can see all the good in you. (7 seconds pause)

164. The path to your future body and weight loss journey is filled with hope and certainty. (7 seconds pause)

165. You are grateful for the body you have and its efforts in helping you through you fat losing pursuit. (7 seconds pause)

166. There are new friends in your life who are going through the same struggles and fights as you. (7 seconds pause)

167. You are a strong, healthy being. (7 seconds pause)

168. Perfecting you're eating habits is becoming easier every day. (7 seconds pause)

169. Your self-confidence is now on the seventh sky with the changes you've made on this journey. (7 seconds pause)

170. Your body deserves your utmost respect and you are taking care of it. (7 seconds pause)

171. It feels great to reside in this new and improved body. (7 seconds pause)

172. You push through all the tough times that come your way because you believe in yourself. (7 seconds pause)

173. You are open to all the best techniques that will help you achieve your ideal body weight. (7 seconds pause)

174. You are discovering that you have an athletic side as well. (7 seconds pause)

175. Day by day, your body is becoming slender and svelte. (7 seconds pause)

176. All your intuitions to judge or critique your body are now buried down in your mind (7 seconds pause)

177. You are fit for life. (7 seconds pause)

178. You love your health. (7 seconds pause)

179. You love the gym. (7 seconds pause)

180. You love exercising. (7 seconds pause)

181. You feel like you are powerful even in and outside the gym. (7 seconds pause)

182. The dreams of weight loss is what you eat, drink, think, walk and talk. (7 seconds pause)

183. You are a strong example of someone who sticks to their goal of weight loss through all highs and lows. (7 seconds pause)

184. This journey has taught you to find humor and joy constantly. (7 seconds pause)

185. You are proud of the progress you made and how far you've come in your weight loss journey. (7 seconds pause)

186. You recognize your efforts verbally and non-verbally everyday. (7 seconds pause)

187. You are looking to participate in new active things to help your journey. (7 seconds pause)

188. Food items that are empty in calories and do not help your health are of no interest to you any longer. (7 seconds pause)

189. You are now a judge of your own habits and eliminate anything that sabotages your weight loss journey. (7 seconds pause)

190. You friends and family are always going to check on you and encourage you to keep working on your weight. (7 seconds pause)

191. You feel no shame when you tell people your goals. You just feel like you have reinforced them a bit more. (7 seconds pause)

192. You give healthy nutrients to your body by eating healthy foods (7 seconds pause)

193. You are full of energy and vitality (7 seconds pause)
194. You love to exercise because it makes you happy (7 seconds pause)
195. You release weight easily and effortlessly (7 seconds pause)
196. You are open to change (7 seconds pause)
197. You let go of the past easily (7 seconds pause)
198. You are waking up feeling happy and energetic everyday (7 seconds pause)
199. You pay attention to your sleep (7 seconds pause)
200. You are strong and healthy (7 seconds pause)
201. You drink at least eight glasses of water everyday (7 seconds pause)
202. You are motivated to exercise every day. (7 seconds pause)
203. You listen to the signal and stop when you have eaten enough (7 seconds pause)
204. You are happy and healthy (7 seconds pause)
205. You love to exercise everyday (7 seconds pause)
206. You love to eat fruits and vegetables everyday (7 seconds pause)
207. You are becoming stronger and slimmer with every passing day (7 seconds pause)
208. You look for natural sugar in fruits (7 seconds pause)
209. You are grateful for your health (7 seconds pause)
210. You are practice gratefulness everyday (7 seconds pause)
211. You are open to new ways of eating and exercising (7 seconds pause)
212. You choose food that make your body stronger and healthier (7 seconds pause)
213. You chew each mouthful at least 8 to 10 times (7 seconds pause)
214. You are becoming slimmer and lighter every day (7 seconds pause)
215. Your body and mind are working harmoniously with each other (7 seconds pause)
216. You enjoy taking care of your body and mind (7 seconds pause)
217. You limit your day time naps to 30 minutes (7 seconds pause)
218. You can do it (7 seconds pause)
219. You are flexible and love your body (7 seconds pause)
220. You listen to your body (7 seconds pause)
221. You eat in moderation and sleep really well every night (7 seconds pause)
222. You eat wholesome foods (7 seconds pause)
223. You leave your past behind (7 seconds pause)
224. You feel enthusiastic (7 seconds pause)
225. You look forward to each day (7 seconds pause)
226. You set everyday sleep and weight loss goals (7 seconds pause)
227. You take everyday actions to achieve goals (7 seconds pause)
228. You are motivated (7 seconds pause)
229. You focus on the good and the glass half full (7 seconds pause)
230. You are grateful to god for all the good things you have in your life(7 seconds pause)
231. You are losing weight with every passing day (7 seconds pause)
232. You are self-aware and aware of your emotions and thoughts (7 seconds pause)
233. You love the taste of healthy food (7 seconds pause)
234. You are grateful for the foods that make you healthy (7 seconds pause)
235. All the weights and burdens from the past are melting away (7 seconds pause)

236.   You are getting lighter and leaner (7 seconds pause)
237.   You are getting fitter and slimmer (7 seconds pause)
238.   You see beauty in your body and appreciate it (7 seconds pause)
239.   You learn new ways easily (7 seconds pause)
240.   Your body is getting healed and you are becoming fitter (7 seconds pause)
241.   Every day you wake up you have feelings of gratitude (7 seconds pause)
242.   You trust the process of life (7 seconds pause)
243.   You trust yourself and trust your body (7 seconds pause)
244.   You love yourself and trust yourself fully (7 seconds pause)
245.   You are compassionate towards yourself (7 seconds pause)
246.   You eat mindfully and enjoy every mouthful (7 seconds pause)
247.   You are competent and capable. (7 seconds pause)
248.   You are worthy of love and care (7 seconds pause)
249.   You give all the love and care to your own body first (7 seconds pause)
250.   You choose positive thoughts and take positive actions (7 seconds pause)
251.   You are blessed and abundant (7 seconds pause)
252.   You love yourself unconditionally and take positive actions eeryday to live your day fully. (7 seconds pause)
253.   You are complete and whole. (7 seconds pause)
254.   You are confident and courageous (7 seconds pause)
255.   You forgive yourself for all the past mistakes (7 seconds pause)
256.   You stay in present and are mindful (7 seconds pause)
257.   You are confident (7 seconds pause)
258.   You are losing weight every day (7 seconds pause)
259.   You are focused on your weight loss journey (7 seconds pause)
260.   You pay attention to your food intake (7 seconds pause)
261.   You chew your food many times (7 seconds pause)
262.   You maintain sleep hygiene (7 seconds pause)
263.   You love yourself unconditionally (7 seconds pause)
264.   Your body is getting fitter and slimmer (7 seconds pause)
265.   You are successful (7 seconds pause)
266.   You are confident and motivated (7 seconds pause)
267.   You believe in yourself (7 seconds pause)
268.   You are good enough (7 seconds pause)
269.   You enjoy healthy foods (7 seconds pause)
270.   You do pleasurable activities everyday (7 seconds pause)
271.   You are intelligent and wise (7 seconds pause)
272.   You are lovable, open to receive and give love (7 seconds pause)
273.   You enjoy your life (7 seconds pause)
274.   You enjoy healthy food (7 seconds pause)
275.   You have a beautiful relationship with food and your body (7 seconds pause)
276.   You are becoming slimmer and stronger (5 seconds Pause)

277.   You are mindful of eating (Same as above)

278.   You exercise regularly (Same as above)

279.   You sleep well every night and take at least 6 hours of deep sleep (Same as above)

280.   You enjoy eating green, dark leafy vegetables (Same as above)

281.   Your body is becoming slimmer with every passing day (Same as above)

282.   You are in control of your life (Same as above)

283.   You have taken charge of your life and body (Same as above)

284.   You feel good when you eat healthy and exercise regularly (Same as above)

285.   Your body gets rid of extra fat (Same as above)

286.   Your love yourself with every passing day (Same as above)

287.   You are motivated to achieve your ideal goal weight (Same as above)

288.   You avoid high calorie food (Same as above)
289.   You enjoy smaller portions of food (Same as above)

290.   You chew eat mouthful atleast 10 times and relish the flavors (Same as above)

291.   You eat fresh fruits and savor the flavors (Same as above)

292.   You look forward to your exercise session every day (Same as above)

293.   You are positive (Same as above)

294.   You are focused on your daily actions and daily goals (Same as above)

295.   You see yourself having the ideal body and weight (Same as above)

296.   You stay focused on this weight loss journey (Same as above)

297.   You enjoy the taste of fresh fruits (Same as above)

298.   You enjoy the taste of veggies (Same as above)

299.   You include lean proteins and skimmed milk in your diet (Same as above)

300.   You enjoy the taste of salads (Same as above)

301. Your body is becoming slimmer (Same as above)

302. Your stomach and hips are becoming smaller (Same as above)

303. You are getting stronger and leaner (Same as above)

304. You gain muscle and lose weight (Same as above)

305. You feel stronger and stronger with every passing day (Same as above)

306. Your trust your body and it gets easier and easier to trust it (Same as above)

307. Your health is improving with every passing day (Same as above)
308. Making small changes are becoming so much easier for you (Same as above)

309. You are patient and believe in yourself (Same as above)

310. You believe that you will achieve the weight loss goal (Same as above)

311. Letting go of past is easier (Same as above)

312. You are in control of your emotions (Same as above)

313. You are focused and determined (Same as above)

314. You are full of energy (Same as above)

315. You are the creator of your own future (Same as above)

316. You believe your strengths and capabilities (Same as above)

317. You are capable to lose weight (Same as above)

318. You love and accept yourself (Same as above)

319. You are full of self-love (Same as above)

320. You give your body all the nutrients it needs (Same as above)

321. Every day of exercise and eating right food makes you even more confident (Same as above)

322. You are confident (Same as above)

323. You have high self-worth (Same as above)

324. Your love for yourself increases with every passing day (Same as above)

325. You are focused on your weight loss journey (Same as above)

326. You are in control of how much you eat (7 seconds pause)
327. You deserve to feel happy and look great (7 seconds pause)
328. You enjoy exercising (7 seconds pause)
329. You eat only when you are hungry (7 seconds pause)
330. You are getting slimmer every day (7 seconds pause)
331. You choose to eat right (7 seconds pause)
332. You deserve to be healthier and attractive (7 seconds pause)
333. You love your body and care for it (7 seconds pause)
334. You are developing healthy eating habits (7 seconds pause)
335. You are happy exercising (7 seconds pause)
336. You are reaching your ideal goal weight soon (7 seconds pause)
337. You eat smaller portions (7 seconds pause)
338. You drink 8 to 10 glasses of water everyday (7 seconds pause)
339. You eat fruits and vegetables and enjoy eating them (7 seconds pause)
340. You celebrate your life and healthy choices (7 seconds pause)
341. You have a flat stomach (7 seconds pause)
342. You are getting attractive and even more charming with every passing day (7 seconds pause)
343. You take charge of your life and body (7 seconds pause)
344. You fall asleep every night effortlessly (7 seconds pause)
345. You love and appreciate your body (7 seconds pause)
346. You love changing your body (7 seconds pause)
347. Your metabolism is faster than before (7 seconds pause)
348. You are mindful and live every moment (7 seconds pause)
349. You are lovable (7 seconds pause)
350. You are a beautiful person (7 seconds pause)
351. You love yourself unconditionally (7 seconds pause)
352. You are complete and whole. (7 seconds pause)
353. You are confident and courageous (7 seconds pause)
354. You forgive yourself for all the past mistakes (7 seconds pause)
355. You stay in present and are more mindful (7 seconds pause)
356. You are confident (7 seconds pause)
357. You have high self-esteem (7 seconds pause)
358. You are losing weight every day (7 seconds pause)
359. You are focused on your weight loss journey (7 seconds pause)
360. You pay attention to your food intake (7 seconds pause)
361. You chew your food many times (7 seconds pause)
362. You maintain sleep hygiene (7 seconds pause)

363. You love yourself unconditionally (7 seconds pause)
364. Your body is getting fitter and slimmer (7 seconds pause)
365. You are successful (7 seconds pause)
366. You are confident and motivated (7 seconds pause)
367. You believe in yourself (7 seconds pause)
368. You are good enough (7 seconds pause)
369. You enjoy healthy foods (7 seconds pause)
370. You do pleasurable activities everyday (7 seconds pause)
371. You are intelligent and wise (7 seconds pause)
372. You are lovable, open to receive and give love (7 seconds pause)
373. You enjoy your life (7 seconds pause)
374. You enjoy healthy food (7 seconds pause)
375. You have a beautiful relationship with food and your body (7 seconds pause)
376. You have a lot of love and approval for yourself. (7 seconds pause)
377. You are at peace with yourself in your body, heart and soul. (7 seconds pause)
378. As each day passes, you feel that you are healthier and stronger inside. (7 seconds pause)
379. Every day, you are learning how to love and appreciate your body. (7 seconds pause)
380. Being yourself is the safest way for you to be. (7 seconds pause)
381. You focus on all the good that is happening in your life. (7 seconds pause)
382. It becomes easier and easier for you to trust your body. (7 seconds pause)
383. You can feel your body and mind getting healed. (7 seconds pause)
384. You are choosing to take in breaths of relaxation and breathe out all your stress. (7 seconds pause)
385. Your health and your life are moving in the direction of improvement. (7 seconds pause)
386. A healing white light surrounds you and is protecting you. (7 seconds pause)
387. Your entire food intake is nourishing your body and healing it well. (7 seconds pause)
388. Every baby step you take is getting you closer to your ideal goal weight. (7 seconds pause)
389. You progress comes above any perfection for you. (7 seconds pause)
390. Your intuition is your guiding light and helps you decide what to eat and how to live your life. (7 seconds pause)
391. You are naturally connecting with like-minded people who bring in positivity. (7 seconds pause)
392. It is best for you to let go of your past. Letting go of the past is safe for you now. (7 seconds pause)
393. You can feel the beginning of changes in everything around you. (7 seconds pause)
394. You are now focused, determined and healthy. (7 seconds pause)
395. You choose for yourself to be slim and healthy. (7 seconds pause)
396. You can see new doors opening in your life with a lot of new and exciting things. (7 seconds pause)
397. You have the ability to heal your body. You are healing your body. (7 seconds pause)
398. You can do this and so you are doing this. Your body is healing right now. (7 seconds pause)
399. A higher power is guiding you along your way. (7 seconds pause)

400. You are a strong, energetic person. (7 seconds pause)
401. You choose to see the best in everyone and so do they. (7 seconds pause)
402. You have faith in your ability of self-love. (7 seconds pause)
403. You truly love yourself for however you are. (7 seconds pause)
404. You have accepted and acknowledged your body shape and the beauty hidden in it.
405. You are the creator of your future. (7 seconds pause)
406. You have now moved on from the unhealthy, unhelpful behavioral pattern around food. (7 seconds pause)
407. The choices and decisions you make for yourself are for your higher good. (7 seconds pause)
408. You are no longer holding on to any regrets or guilt about your past food choices. (7 seconds pause)
409. You have accepted your body's shape and you feel blessed for what you have. (7 seconds pause)
410. You have moved farther away from relationships that don't contribute to your betterment. (7 seconds pause)
411. You acknowledge your own greatness. (7 seconds pause)
412. You allow yourself to feel good about being you. (7 seconds pause)
413. You have an acceptance for yourself. (7 seconds pause)
414. You are letting in the qualities of love in your heart. (7 seconds pause)
415. You see your future filled with hope and certainty. (7 seconds pause)
416. You find gratefulness in your heart for your body and all you do for your well-being. (7 seconds pause)
417. You indulge in a healthy amount of exercise on a regular basis. (7 seconds pause)
418. Your body is getting all the nutrients that it requires. (7 seconds pause)
419. You are developing a strong urge to eat food that is nutritious (7 seconds pause)
420. You feel good about yourself. (7 seconds pause)
421. You are on your way to attaining and maintaining your ideal weight. (7 seconds pause)
422. You are a strong, healthy person. (7 seconds pause)
423. You are now peaceful and calm. (7 seconds pause)
424. The Universe has gifted you with your mind, body and soul. (7 seconds pause)
425. Your body is your temple (7 seconds pause)
426. You love your body and take care of it every single day.. (7 seconds pause)
427. Everyday imagine yourself looking in the Victorian mirror to meet your ideal self at the ideal goal weight. (7 seconds pause)
428. You love your body just the way it is and you know you can make it better only when you accept it fully. (7 seconds pause)
429. You are grateful everyday for the nutritious food, every breath, your house, and your family. (7 seconds pause)
430. You are grateful for all the positive and good things in life. (7 seconds pause)
431. You appreciate your life and appreciate your body (7 seconds pause)
432. You love yourself even more (7 seconds pause)
433. You enjoy losing weight (7 seconds pause)
434. You try clothes every week to see how well they fit you (7 seconds pause)
435. Life is good for you (7 seconds pause)
436. You are excited and look forward to every day (7 seconds pause)

437.   You live your day productively (7 seconds pause)
438.   You have a fulfilling life (7 seconds pause)

All these suggestions are firmly embedded in your sub-conscious mind and with every passing day, getting stronger and stronger with every passing day, hour, minute.

Waking Up

In a moment, I am going to count you up from one to five and with each count up, you will be back in the present moment and wide awake. Feeling fully refreshed and looking forward to the new you.

Starting now at one, two, three, coming slowly back, four – eyelids beginning to flutter and five – eyes open wide awake.

Gastric Band Hypnosis: Beginners Guided & Self-Hypnosis For Weight Loss, Burning Fat, Overcoming Food Addiction, Eating Healthy Including Positive Affirmations & Meditations

By Meditation Made Effortless

Table of Contents

To the Narrator

The Introduction, Induction, and Deepener should be 45 Min Long

Hypnotic Gastric Band should be 30 Min long

Eat smaller portions should be 20 Min long

Develop self-love should be 25 Min long

Overcome junk food cravings 30 Min

should be 25 min long

Stop emotional eating should be 15 min long

Ego strengthening script should be 25 min long

More weight loss should be 15 min long

Weight object of the past should be 30 min long

Reinforcement Script should be 20 min long

Affirmations – should be 50 min long

"..." means take a breath while speaking before you continue.

PAUSE (for a few breaths)

LONGER PAUSE (give time to allow the listener time to imagine what you've suggested)

Introduction

Thank you for choosing **Gastric Band Hypnosis audio**...And choosing this audio only means, you have taken a step towards loving yourself even more. In the past, you may have gained weight because of many reasons and you are aware of that. You are also aware that it is important to lose extra weight and have a fitter and healthier body. That is why you are listening to this audio. Isn't it?

Hypnotic gastric band also called as virtual gastric band will allow you to believe that your stomach has shrunk to a size of a golf ball and because of that it can take in smaller amounts of food. You will believe that your stomach is a size of a golf ball and you will eat accordingly exactly how people eat when they get the expensive invasive gastric band surgery done.

Listening to this audio means that you have agreed to believe that your stomach is going to be much smaller in size and that will help you shed extra weight much faster.

When you listen to this recording every day, you reinforce that you are on a weight loss journey where your stomach has shrunken to a size of a golf ball allowing you to eat much lesser, boosting your metabolism, and ultimately helping you lose all the extra weight.

Pause

So, congratulations on taking this step to undergo hypnotic gastric band procedure. Every time you listen to this audio, you get more and more focused on knowing that your stomach has shrunken to a size of a golf ball, you have a band fitted on your stomach, and you eat smaller portions.

Pause

I would like you to sit or lay comfortably, where you will not be distracted. Do not listen to this audio when your mind requires your conscious attention.

Pause

Listen to this audio only when you are relaxed and stationary. Please use headphones so that you can focus on the sound of my voice.

Let us start...

Begin recording

Induction

You are now listening to the sound of my voice... and the sound of my voice only ...and as you continue to listen to each word I say...you allow yourself to relax more and more.

Pause

I wonder if you could take a deep breath...hold it for a count of 5... and then exhale.

Pause

Let's start now.

Breathe in Deeply...

Pause

Hold for a count of 5

1... 2...3...4...and 5

Now, exhale...

Pause

Once more, take another deep breath...

Breathe in...

Hold for a count of 5 — 1, 2, 3, 4, 5 (slowly)

Now, breathe out...

Pause

Once more, take another deep breath —

Breathe in

Hold for a count of 5 — 1, 2, 3, 4, 5 (slowly)

Now, breathe out

Pause

And, come back to your normal breathing pattern...

Pause

— And, I wonder... if you could simply bring all your focus and attention to the centre of your eye-brows...with your eyes closed...try to look at the centre of your brows and focus on the point between them...that's right.

Pause

In a moment, I am going to talk to that part of you, which is highly creative...the part that knows exactly how to help you imagine or create anything with the help of your mind's eye.

Pause

And... I know you can do it... because everybody can...we all have a creative mind, that has the ability and capability to create and imagine images in our mind.

I know you must have imagined or visualized or day-dreamed many times in your life. And... our creative part helps us imagine and visualize. Isn't it?

With the help of our creative mind, we can visualize, imagine, write, paint, and dream...and I am going to be talking to that part of you today.

Pause

Deepener

And I wonder if you can imagine or visualize that you are somewhere in a luxury beach resort. And as soon as you enter, you can smell the lovely fragrance at the entrance.

You wonder what scent is that...

The staff caters to your every need and you feel truly pampered and cared for.

In the room of the luxury resort, you notice a beautiful lounger in the patio that overlooks the beautiful sea waters...the lounger has a comfy cushion on it and is perhaps made of sturdy wood. The lounger is tilting a bit backwards for you to relax on it and enjoy the beautiful surroundings. You take a seat and rest your arms on the chair's hand rests.

Pause

You notice the beautiful sun shining and the green tall palm trees swaying with the sea breeze. Far away, you look at the horizon and the many sailboats...perhaps there are 5 or more...

You continue to enjoy the surroundings and enjoy this time alone...so calm and serene.

In a moment, you feel the Sunshine over you and it feels nice and warm...you cover your face with a hat and put the Sun tan lotion all over your body ...and you let yourself soak up the Sun.

Pause

You are all alone here in your room's large patio and there are no people around. You only listen to the sound of the waves and perhaps the sound of the seagulls.

You decide to close your eyes and take a nap...

Pause

And, in a moment, I am going to count you down from 10 down to 0...with each count down, you will be twice as deep and twice as relaxed...

Starting now...

10...relaxing more and more

9...going deeper and deeper

8... into a beautiful state of relaxation

7...allowing yourself to drift down...

5...deeper and deeper...

4...further deep...

3...all your body parts are getting relaxed...

2...even more relaxed...

1...deeper and deeper...

0 – Deep Sleep

Hypnotic Gastric Band Procedure

And as you continue to listen to me...I wonder if you can let go and simply relax your mind and body...for you to easily access your mind's creative part...

A part of you is creative and it allows you to imagine things from the eyes of your mind.

Longer Pause

And I wonder if you can let your creative part help you imagine that you are

entering a door having a long corridor at the end of it -

Somewhere inside your heart...you know that you are entering a procedural room where gastric band procedure will be done. -

Pause

And now slowly and slowly...move towards the door-

You are already aware that this is the safest and renowned place for conducting the procedure -

You trust the doctors and staff...

You already know a lot of people that have lost weight and followed up with the doctors for further consultation here...

You have seen a lot of successful people who have lost so much weight with the help of gastric band, fitted on their stomachs.

Now you must be feeling more confident about this procedure...isn't it?

You believe this will be successful and by the end of the procedure...you stomach would have shrunk to a size of a golf ball.

Longer Pause

The time to enter the clinic is here.

And you push open the door...and enter the clinic...

You are feeling nice about the decision you have made while you enter the clinic

It feels great when you think about the decision taken to go to a procedure involving gastric band

This contracts your stomach...you start feeling full...which in turn results to, you having smaller amounts of food...this way your metabolism increases helping you in losing weight and the ideal goal weight becomes much easier to achieve...

Pause

This is a time of immense happiness for you as today...you have taken a step towards your new version and you have decided to lose weight that has been a a long time desire...isn't it?

Pause

You are now heading towards the procedure room-

You feel relaxed on seeing the staff around you.

You have already booked an appointment with the doctor a week before and you know that the staff is skilled...and they will take good care...

The nurse reminds you that, when they put a silicone band around the stomach...it restricts the food intake which helps in eating less leading you to lose weight easily...

You have a full trust in yourself and the procedure.

Pause

The band will contract it and make it much smaller so that you can take in smaller amounts of foods.

The size would be as small as a golf ball...

It will help in much faster weight loss...

Pause

You will lose weight faster when you consume less food ensuring lesser calorie intake and faster metabolism.

Pause

You might start to think that you are entering a procedural room and that makes you feel calmer and safe...

You are in safe hands...you trust the doctors and nurses...

Pause

As the time passes and the staff talks to you in a friendly way...you feel more and more relaxed...

And in a moment, you notice that you are drifting away into a dream like state while the doctors talk to you about your life...and the sounds of their voices fade away...

You are drifting further and further into a dream like state...a beautiful state of relaxation...and as you enter the deepest state of hypnosis...with your mind's eye...you notice the color of your stomach...

Pause

Perhaps it's either pink or brown...get the knowing of the color of your stomach...

You see it in a particular size...and in a moment...you know that the size of your stomach would reduce when the gastric band will be fitted...

And you are looking forward to the procedure...

You are excited...for this change...the change that will make you feel much better about yourself and much more confident about your body...

Pause

You see that a band is being placed around your stomach...right on top it...making your stomach look really small...

You are closely looking at its size...

And when you observe the size you know that you can only eat much smaller portions of food...

With the gastric band, you can eat food without any diet plans...you only have to eat smaller portions of healthy and nutritious food...and I know you can do it...because everybody can...

Pause

The band is tightly fitted on the top of your stomach and it stays there for a long time...

You feel much fuller because of the silicone band and you consume food at a slower pace...

The procedure is complete.

Longer Pause

You are free from scars as the procedure has been successfully performed by professional doctors...

Indeed successful...

From now on...your stomach size has been reduced to a size of a golf ball...and it can only accommodate smaller portions of food...that's right...

With this band on your stomach, you will lose weight effortlessly..

Pause

To make the process of digestion faster, you chew food 8 to 12 times...enjoying the flavors of the food...

You are mindful of what you eat and you enjoy each mouthful...

Everyday...you get to feel that your stomach has contracted to the size of a golf ball...and it can take in smaller amounts of food only...

Pause

The procedure is complete...and it has been a success...

You come out of the procedural room...take the discharge slip...the next day...and go back home, feeling absolutely excited for the results that follow...

Imagine being at your goal weight now...

See yourself enjoying what you would enjoy by being at the goal weight...

Longer Pause

I wonder if you can now repeat the following suggestions in your mind after me...

I love consuming smaller portions every day

I feel confident

I make a conscious effort to eat less

I chew my food atleast 8 times

I enjoy the flavors of foods

I relish and enjoy each mouthful...

Eat Smaller Portions

As you continue to listen to each word I say...you allow yourself to stay focused on eating less because you know that your stomach can take in lesser amounts of foods only.

A band is now fitted on the top of your stomach and you can see it with your mind's eye...

The hypnotic gastric band has shrunken the size of your stomach which can now only take lesser amounts of foods...

Listen to this audio more often to know and get convinced that your stomach is much smaller now and with every passing day, you need lesser amounts of food and get satisfied with smaller portions of food...

This will ensure that you reach the goal that you have set for yourself – your ideal body weight...

Note that you must always listen to what my voice is saying. Your mind might wander for a few minutes but you should bring it back by paying attention to this audio...

Pause

You are paying attention to the sound of my voice.

While you pay heed to every word of this recording, you are feeling more relaxed...

As you grasp the word that I say, it is indicating that you are ready to absorb whatever I am saying...

You know now that the size of your stomach is very small...and

You have always wanted to lose weight so your stomach has become smaller helping you to lose weight faster.

Your love for yourself has increased now...

You are aware of what your feelings are, how you behave and act... and the way you think.

Eating a small amount of foods helps in increasing your body metabolism...which in turn results in a faster weight loss.

Every time you eat, you chew food more frequently to get the flavors and taste of the food...

You eat food, enjoy it...and fill your small stomach with nutrients...

Pause

With every word of mine, you start believing how easy it is to intake the right amount of food and lose weight...

And, I would like to talk that creative part of your mind again to show you that you are somewhere in grassy fields...

Longer Pause

The sun is shining bright...

You can smell the smell the fresh air...

Pause

You are in a big magnificent field...

This sunshine is making the field look beautiful and bright...

You feel relaxed as you sit on the ground...

I am wondering if you have ever thought of the reasons why you want to lose weight and get slimmer.

Pause

Are you imagining yourself at your desired weight and size?

Try to get that picture into your mind.

Pause

You are wearing the clothes that you always wanted to wear.

Think of yourself as a person who is much more confident and has high self-esteem.

Pause

How are you feeling about this new weight, what are your body expressions telling you about your new weight and size?

It's time to conceive your actions and your feelings.

You have an inbuilt feeling imbibed in you that makes you realize what is the maximum that you can bear. You will feel that you had sufficient food.

When you get a feeling that you are full, you automatically stop. Sometimes you leave the food on your plate too when you get a feeling that your stomach can't take more.

Pause

It's the time to enter your brain through your imaginative mind.

It is the time to enter your brain, look for a button that signals that your stomach is full.

Start imagining and feel that you are entering your brain.

You are aware that it is your brain that is the governing factor.

It is the time to get inside your brain and look for that particular button

You overeat only when your button does not function well indicating wrong signals, it is the time to get it fixed.

You can only lose weight if the gastric band is in the right place and you are eating less.

You can fix the button so that it functions well and start indicating that the stomach is full.

Pause

The stomach is now of the same size as that of the golf ball.

Longer Pause

You have succeeded in fixing it.

You must check if the button has started working well, indicating the brain that it is the right time to stop eating.

Pause

Now that the button has started functioning giving you the right signals

Start imagining yourself seated in a chair having a table placed in front of you.

The table has a small plate filled with food

Pause

You look towards your plate and eat only that much amount which is ideal for your stomach which has a reduced capacity now

You drink water before eating food

Now you start eating food by gradual chewing and then repeat the step for 15 to 20 times...enjoying the taste and flavours

Pause

Your stomach has reduced in size...so you intake only small amounts of food

Every time you take more food to fill up your plate...you automatically get a signal from the brain and then you stop

That's right

Pause

After you know that you have eaten a lot of food...you just stop

You drink a glass of water after finishing your food...

Every day you feel that your stomach is shrinking and you are getting slimmer by eating small amounts of food...eventually leading to a boost in your metabolism.

You drink at least 8 glasses of water everyday —

Sometimes, you make the water taste good by putting in some lemon or mint...

Every time you eat food, you remember your future image at the target goal weight...

You are aware that if you intake a small amount then you will accomplish your desired goal very soon.

Pause

Every meal boosts up your confidence and energizes you by making you feel confident

From now on...you eat smaller meals...and frequent meals...

Pause

You like small means now (7-8 seconds of pause)

You chew the food atleast 8 to 10 times… (7-8 seconds of pause)

You look ahead for a new to accomplish your goal much sooner (7-8 seconds of pause)

You start feeling grateful about yourself (7-8 seconds of pause)

You stay energized all day by eating small amounts of food (7-8 seconds of pause)

You are much happier and active now (7-8 seconds of pause)

You will be conscious of the amount that you eat from today (7-8 seconds of pause)

You have around 8 glasses of water (7-8 seconds of pause)

Toxins will be released on drinking water and weight loss will be accelerated (7-8 seconds of pause)

You experience faster weight loss (7-8 seconds of pause)

You see a new version of yourself-slimmer, fitter, and happy (7-8 seconds of pause)

You have realized when to stop eating food by sensing how full is your stomach (7-8 seconds of pause)

And as you continue to lose weight and look fitter…I wonder what everyone around you is saying…

Are they proud of what you have achieved?

Longer Pause

Develop Self Love / Inner Child

And I wonder if you can imagine a hallway somewhere…and imagine that hallway leading you to a door…and the door leads you to a garden.

Pause

And, in a moment, you walk towards the door through the hallway…to see how the garden looks like…and it is going to be a beautiful place…

You are now at the door…you touch the door and feel its texture…perhaps its old or new… and in a moment you push open it…

Longer Pause

And as you push open it…you find yourself surrounded by a beautiful garden…

You are in a garden…the garden looks beautiful…and you see many bushes and trees, and feel the lush green grass beneath your feet. As you look around you notice that the garden is magically beautiful with flowers in the bushes…

And as you look further around, you notice a child who looks exactly like how you used to look like when you were young.

Longer Pause

You are amused to see the child and you walk over to the child…the child is sitting on a bench in the garden…

You look at the child and look at the clothes…the shoes…the hair….and the child looks adorable.

You go to the child and give them a big hug…and as that happens the child feels safe and gets into your lap and smiles back.

You tell the child – you are adorable and I love you unconditionally

I love you for who you are and I am proud of you.

You also say that I am sorry for coming to see you after so many years…I am really sorry if I have hurt you ever…I love you and truly do.

Longer Pause

You tell the child that how special he or she is to you…and in a while, you begin to play with the child.

And as you start to play with each other…you begin to enjoy the beautiful bond

That you have with your inner child…its amazing to be in touch with it…isn't it. Together…as you continue to play…you feel and notice that the bond is strengthening…

Pause

And as you both continue to play with each other…the child gets even more comfy with you and comes back in your arms and lap…trusting you even more…

In a moment...you will notice the child integrating into you...and as that happens, you notice...that the child becomes one with you...and you embrace the child...just the way the child is...

Pause

In a moment, as I count from 3 down to 0, with each count down...you notice the child coming closer and then integrating into you...making you whole and complete...as one individual full of self-love...and this only means...that you allow yourself to love even more...

Pause

When it comes to weight loss...you are focused on the path you have chosen to see yourself as fitter, slimmer, and happier....

You are whole and complete...completely focused on achieving your ideal goal weight...and that would be possible if you love yourself completely and unconditionally...

Overcome Junk Food Cravings

And you focus on the sound of my voice and the sound of my voice only...and as you listen to each word I say...you allow yourself to go deeper and deeper and be more and more receptive to what I am saying...

Pause

You know that all your feelings are valid and they are there for a reason. They let you take a certain action so that you are in charge of your life...exactly like how we live in a house and we have electricity, water, power, and kitchen helping us to know what is needed to keep everything going.

Pause

In the same way, our feelings are like electricity, water, power, kitchen, backyard...that allow us to know what is happening to our body and we can take charge of it and take care of ourselves.

Pause

In the same way, by listening to your feelings, you can take care of your body better. If you treat your house the way you have been treating your body...then what would happen?

Perhaps the kitchen groceries would run out of stock if you don't pay attention to the stock or if you do not mow the grass in your backyard or front lawn, you may have overgrown grass and it would perhaps look unkept and ugly...

Longer Pause

And, when you pay attention...you can control everything and take charge of your house.

Similarly, to keep the body working aptly in the best condition, you need to keep attending to the feelings and take actions accordingly for your body's highest good.

If you feel anxious, the action you need to take is to calm yourself down or do a mindful exercise rather than moving towards food and filling yourself up with junk that will make you feel guilty once you have finished eating.

Pause

Another feeling could be stress and it means you have too much on your plate and you are trying to finish everything in a certain amount of time...but instead of turning towards eating junk...you need to look for ways to reduce stress.

Pause

Similarly, you may have many feelings ...but that needs your action to resolve and feel better rather than turning to food and then feel guilty.

From today on, you will be able to pay attention to the feelings and take right actions that allow you to resolve the issue without turning to food.

Longer Pause

You worship your body and in no way you can allow it to get ruined by eating rut or junk food. Junk food is high on sugar and it may give you pleasure temporarily but you know the long-term ill effects of it...isn't it?

And I wonder if you know how eating junk food can affect your cardiovascular health...because they are high in saturated fat, it increases the bad cholesterol in your blood that puts your heart functioning at risk. With too much salt, you may have an increase in high blood pressure, again may put your heart at risk.

Pause

And when it comes to gaining weight, the big culprit is junk food, which is high in calories, sugar, and salt content...and eating junk food three times a week can lead you to gain 1 pound in just about one week.

And, I wonder if you can imagine that you continue to eat junk food for another three months....

Just imagine that now...

Longer Pause

And, you do not have to be like that...you can start the change from today on and instead of junk food, you snack on fruits, vegetables, wheat crackers, fat free dressings and make delicious salads.

You are ready to have a healthy lifestyle with food that is more satisfying than all the rut that you have been eating...

And when any feeling comes, you know how to tackle it exactly how you tackle things at home to keep the home running perfectly...isn't it?

Longer Pause

When you are feeling emotionally or mentally hungry…you divert your thoughts by first showing a "stop signal" to your thought and then distract yourself to resolve the negative feeling in a better way…

And, then when you are physically hungry, you eat healthy food…food that is tasty and healthier…whole grains, lentils, milk, fruits, vegetables…you eat all of this to slim down, look better, and feel amazing…

I know you can do it…because everybody can…

Affirmations

I would like you to now repeat the following in your mind:

- I enjoy eating healthy food
- I am in control of your emotions and actions
- I love myself
- I see myself at my ideal goal weight
- I enjoy eating healthy foods
- I love eating fruits and vegetables and whole grains
- I exercise every day for at least 30 minutes

Stop Emotional Eating

And you continue to focus on the sound of my voice and the sound of my voice only...and this only means you allow yourself to be more receptive to what I am saying...

Your subconscious is very powerful and creative and you will allow your subconscious to show you that a beautiful white light surrounds you from all sides.

You notice the light, perhaps it's the light from the land of the supreme power or whoever you believe in...or perhaps it's your own light of unconditional love and purity...

And it begins to surround you from all sides and enters every part of your body, every cell, fiber, bone and nerve...that's right.

Imagine that happening now...

Longer Pause

And as you continue to feel the lovely white light inside and outside of you...you begin to feel safe...and loved.

That's right...

And, in a moment...you notice yourself on a path in a valley...with grassy fields on both sides...and there is a hill you notice in front of you...with a hill top that is shining bright because of the Sunshine...

Pause

You...continue to walk on the path...as you continue to enjoy the surroundings and how you feel looking at all the scenic beauty...perhaps there is a water stream somewhere...the gorgeous trees, the fragrance of moss and flowers, butterflies on the bushes, and birds in the trees...hopping from one branch to another...

You notice the natural beauty and you keep walking forward...

And as you walk...you do feel...and you feel tired...and you wonder what makes you feel tired...

Longer Pause

And as you think about what makes you feel tired...you notice your coat...and you are perhaps feeling tired because of the old rugged coat that you have on...which makes you feel tired and you are unable to walk fast...it drags you down...it makes you tired...

And I wonder why...

Pause

As you look at your coat, you notice that it is old with many pockets...two front pockets and two side pockets...and they are full of some old stuff and clutter...

And you want to reach the hill top to enjoy the birds eye view of the valley...you want to reach the top, the ideal top, the goal is to be there...to be at your ideal weight...

And, I know you can do it...because everybody can...

Pause

You put your hands inside the pockets...and you notice...old papers and stones with many things written on them...that people may have told you knowingly or unknowingly and caused you emotional pain...

And because you have been carrying these in your coat....it makes you feel heavy and tired...and you can barely move forward...

Pause

You know you cannot let your past drive your present...it cannot make you feel heavy, fat, and tired...

The time has come to get rid of the coat now.

Longer Pause

And, I wonder if you can discard the coat somewhere in your valley before you move forward and reach the hill top...

Longer Pause

You have gotten rid of the old heavy rugged coat...and as soon as you have taken if off...you feel free...

You feel light...and energetic...

You are excited to reach the hill top by running towards it...

So....run and reach the hill top...that's your goal...and you can achieve any goal if you feel happy, energetic, and free from the past...

Longer Pause

In a moment you see yourself on the hill top...as someone who is freer, lighter, and happier...

That's right...

Ego Strengthening Script

And as you continue to listen to me and allow yourself to be more receptive and continue to drift deeper and deeper...

You have decided and are fully ready to make significant changes to your body and life to make it even happier and fulfilling.

Pause

And with every word you hear, you become fully aware of the times in the past that made you feel confident and good about yourself. This could be a time from teenage or yearly adulthood...

Get the knowing of that time now...

And as you think about those situations, I wonder if you can choose one that made you feel amazing, happy, confident, and made you believe in your worth.

Longer Pause

And, now that you think of that incident...I want you to watch it in your mind...and as you begin to watch it...you begin to watch it from the beginning...from the time the incident started...

And knowing what you did and how it made you feel and what all it made you think about yourself...

Become aware of those positive emotions and thoughts now...

That's right.

Longer Pause

And now you come to the end of it...

The time has come to watch it on a big TV screen...or even bigger...perhaps a projector screen in a room.

And, I wonder if you can imagine watching that good event...which made you feel great about yourself...made you feel confident, happy, and proud...
Imagine that incident being played on a big projector screen and you are sitting on a couch watching it...

You have its controller in your hand...with many buttons on it...

And as you begin to watch it...you increase the volume to the level of 10...

That's right...

And as you continue to watch...you reach that moment which gave you maximum happiness and confidence...

And as you reach there...you zoom in the scene 10 times...

That's right...

Pause

And you can make the colours brighter and vivid...

Its loud, clear, and vivid....

And you take a mental screenshot of this....and store it somewhere in your mind...

Find a place in your mind to keep the screenshot saved.

Longer Pause

And, you know the place where you have stored it...and every time you feel low in life, you simply remind yourself of all the confidence and happiness your past self had achieved...and you can achieve it again...you can show this screenshot to empower your present self...

Longer Pause

And I wonder if you can practice everyday filling yourself with the color of confidence as soon as you wake up...to feel great in the morning and stay with the feeling throughout the day...

So, imagine a color of confidence...that you resonate with...it is different for everyone...

Think of a color that relates to confidence for you.

Pause

And slowly and slowly allow that colour to move into your body from all sides...perhaps starting from head or feet...

Let the colour reach every part of your body, fibre, cell, and bone...

Fill yourself up with the colour of confidence...the confidence that makes you feel happier, energetic, joyful, and positive.

With happiness and confidence, you can achieve your ideal goal weight...it just gets so much easier when you believe in yourself and have high self-esteem and self-worth...

Pause

You know that you have been confident before and you are confident and get even more confident when you practice filling yourself up with the colour of confidence every morning...

The more your practice it the stronger your confidence becomes...

You lose weight when you eat right and exercise to burn off extra calories. This confidence helps you gain control on your eating habits and how you live your life...

And with every passing day, you notice your confidence goes to the next level...

With high level of confidence, it gets easier for you to know the ways to achieve your goal weight. And, with every passing day, your self-esteem and self-worth is increasing....

You think and talk confidently...and its visible in your body language...you exude self confidence in your walk and how you behave with people...your friends and family are amazed to see you talk so confidently...

Longer Pause

You allow yourself to release all the fears and other negative emotions...that serve no purpose...and allow yourself to feel the positive emotions like security, freedom, positivity, happiness, confidence, calmness...contentment...

Pause

You are aligned and centred at all times... always looking at living your present day and living it mindfully to achieve the daily goals...living each day beautifully and productively.

Longer Pause

You maintain calm and relaxed...focused and mindful. You are confident and secure about everything.

Pause

More Weight Loss

And as you continue to listen to each word I say and allow yourself to go deeper and deeper into a beautiful state of relaxation...

You are open to all my suggestions and this audio is designed to keep weight off permanently...so that you become lean, slim, happy, and even more positive person.

Pause

As you listen to this audio, you are reconditioning your mind to become a new person with a leaner and slimmer body having new eating habits.

With new eating habits, you feel empowered and happier and perhaps become a role model for others...by setting such great example.

Pause

You enjoy life and eat only when you are physical hungry and you eat to nurture and nourish your body...and no other time, you eat food.

In the past, you ate more than your body needed and perhaps you ate to satiate your emotional and mental needs. And because you ate more than what was required, you stored this extra energy as fat.

Pause

To burn this extra stored fat, you eat less each day and when you eat less that you require for the storage will make up the difference.

Longer Pause

And, because your stomach is now restricted, you will naturally eat lesser amounts of food and burn the fat faster. And, whatever healthy foods you will eat, you will be able to satisfy your hunger. You eat less and burn fat faster.

When you eat lesser amounts of healthy food, it shows up on your body and face. Your become slimmer and leaner with every passing day and you are amused to see the clothes getting lose on you.

Pause

You look forward to wearing fitter and smarter clothes and this motivates you even more to exercise and eat less.

You are consistently eating lesser amounts of food because your stomach is now shrunken to a size of a golf ball.

And because of this, you eat much lesser portions of food...and you see yourself as more confident person. You are happy with this transformation and your new form.

Pause

And I wonder if you allow these suggestions to sink into your subconscious for the purpose of your highest good. Also...you notice an image of your future slimmer self-flashing in your mind, the self who enjoys eating lesser amounts of nutritious and healthy food.

Longer Pause

And you have a changed mindset now...the mindset that you have enough to eat and you will never be starved. And, because there is plenty of food around you, you eat it when you want to it and how much you want to eat it. You will not hoard food inside you that makes you fat.

You are losing weight faster every day as you make a conscious effort to eat less because you know that your stomach is a size of a golf ball.

Pause

And as you continue to eat lesser amounts of food, you see yourself slimming down and getting into the shape that you desire. The excess weight is coming off...perhaps melting away...and vanishing...

That's right.

You are in complete control of your life...and your eating habits.

Weight Loss – Object of Past

And you continue to listen to me because you have a wonderful goal in your mind to be at your ideal goal weight...

You know that your stomach is now of a golf ball size and can take in much lesser amounts of foods...

And you are excited to achieve the weight loss results because of the gastric band fitted on your stomach...

Pause

You want to achieve you ideal goal weight and when you think every day about your weight, you must only think of it as the thing of past...and the goal of this recording is to help you let go of the weight problem so that your powerful subconscious mind can keep you focused on the road of weight loss for you to achieve a much slimmer and fitter body...looking absolutely stunning and attractive.

That's right...

Pause

And, I wonder if you can think of your weight issue as an object...it could be anything that comes to your mind...

Think of it as an object...and the object is a depiction of not only your weight, the pounds or kilos but also all the causes that led you to gain weight...the old habits of eating excess food and unhealthy food or eating when you were emotionally hungry...

Longer Pause

And all the effects of being overweight...think of all those and see the causes and effects in the object...

And, I wonder if you could give it a color...

And a texture....

Perhaps observe the shape of the object...

And get the knowing of its weight...is it too heavy?

Get the knowing of how this heavy object has made you feel about yourself in the past...

And now imagine what if you did not have to carry this object...how would your life be different?

Longer Pause

So, you now the time has come to put the weight problem down...put the object down...

And as soon as you do that...you feel the sense of calm all around you...and inside of you...

You can notice all the causes and effects of your old weight issue in that object and the time has come to let go of it completely...because it's not solving any purpose...

And you imagine seeing a helium balloon coming down to take this object with it...far away...away from you...away from your body...

The helium balloon comes down with every breath you take and with every word I say...becoming bigger and bigger as it comes closer and closer...

Longer Pause

And in a moment, you notice the balloon attaching itself to the object magically and takes a flight back to the sky with the object...attached to it...

That's right...

You notice it going up and up...far away...and you notice it becoming smaller and smaller because its moving farther and farther away...back to the sky...across the sky...

And as that happens...you start to feel so much lighter...and freer...as you have completely removed the object of weight from your life...

And you can time travel in your future and see how you look six months from now with the gastric band fitted on your stomach...with no weight object...eating healthily and exercising daily...

That's right...

Meet your future self now...and see how your future self greets and meets you...welcoming and accepting...

And, I wonder if you can move into the body of your future self to feel it and feel how your future self feels and thinks at the ideal goal weight...

And as you enter the body of your future self... you can feel the self's strong, slender, and attractive body...

Pause

See what clothes the future self is wearing...

Notice how the future self is talking and walking...is it more confident?

Now, have a heart to heart conversation with the future self and ask for advice and words of wisdom...perhaps the future self has something amazing to share with you that will change your life for good...

Ask what you need to know the most...and you will get all the guidance from your wise future self...

Longer Pause

Make a mental note of the advice and guidance given by the future self..

And with that...you know that the object of weight has gone far away and can never return...all the causes leading to weight gain and the effects have been dissolved...

You can visit your future self anytime and ask for the guidance or just simply meet by closing your eyes and counting down from 10 down to 0...and at 0..you can imagine your future self...

You can do that...anytime to feel motivated to stay on the road to weight loss...and to seek guidance...

That's right...

Reinforcement Script

As you continue to listen to me...and as we tap into your very powerful mind...you are going to have an amazing relationship with yourself...

You are going to understand yourself and your body better...

You will have a changed and better relationship with food...

Pause

You allow yourself to open to only positive thoughts and be absolutely closed to old negative thoughts, beliefs, and negative emotions...arising from past events...

You are in control...the more control you are...the better is your state of mind...with more control... you feel more relaxed...

That's right...

And I wonder if you can imagine yourself standing on top of a staircase and this time...you see yourself a little different...

You see yourself as more in control...feeling calm and relaxed...knowing all your positive qualities and strengths...

Longer Pause

And perhaps at your ideal goal weight...

Get the sense of it...notice how you look, feel, and how you are standing with straight body posture exuding unending confidence.

I am going to count down from 10 down to 0...it reinforces that this is you. Confident, at your ideal goal weight, knowing all your positive qualities...

10...stepping down the staircase

9...

8....

7...strengthening this is you...

6...

5...

4...knowing this is you

3...confident

2...sealing in the image in your subconscious

1...

0...This is You.

You now begin to think of all the reasons you want to lose weight...and the benefits attached to being at the ideal goal weight...

Longer Pause

Perhaps some of the benefits are more energy, good health, fitter and slimmer, feel attractive, more in control, and wear attractive and fashionable clothes...

Maybe you would be more active and energetic...have better sex life...

The list goes on...

Pause

Your subconscious mind which is the powerful and creative mind will find many healthy and creative ways to move your body more...and with every passing day...you are becoming more and more comfortable with the new body image...at your ideal goal weight...With every passing moment... the fact is strengthening that you have achieved your ideal goal weight...and you are well aware of what that brings with it...all the happiness.. Your drive and motivation is to feel happier every day.

Pause

You may find that that your body and mind are harmoniously working together to help you achieve your ideal goal weight...

That's right.

You are more ready than ever to live a fulfilling life...to be aware and conscious of all the good things that life has to offer to you...

Pause

You begin to realize that you can be relaxed and calm...and are in flow with everything that is happening around you...

With every passing day...you are more energetic and more productive...

That's right...

Affirmations

1. You are in control of how much you eat (7 seconds pause)
2. You deserve to feel happy and look great (7 seconds pause)
3. You enjoy exercising (7 seconds pause)
4. You eat only when you are hungry (7 seconds pause)
5. You are getting slimmer every day (7 seconds pause)
6. You choose to eat right (7 seconds pause)
7. You deserve to be healthier and attractive (7 seconds pause)
8. You love your body and care for it (7 seconds pause)
9. You are developing healthy eating habits (7 seconds pause)
10. You are happy exercising (7 seconds pause)
11. You are reaching your ideal goal weight soon (7 seconds pause)
12. You eat smaller portions (7 seconds pause)
13. You drink 8 to 10 glasses of water everyday (7 seconds pause)
14. You eat fruits and vegetables and enjoy eating them (7 seconds pause)
15. You celebrate your life and healthy choices (7 seconds pause)
16. You have a flat stomach (7 seconds pause)
17. You are getting attractive and even more charming with every passing day (7 seconds pause)
18. You take charge of your life and body (7 seconds pause)
19. You fall asleep every night effortlessly (7 seconds pause)
20. You love and appreciate your body (7 seconds pause)
21. You love changing your body (7 seconds pause)
22. Your metabolism is faster than before (7 seconds pause)
23. You are mindful and live every moment (7 seconds pause)
24. You are lovable (7 seconds pause)
25. You are a beautiful person (7 seconds pause)
26. You love yourself unconditionally (7 seconds pause)
27. You are complete and whole. (7 seconds pause)
28. You are confident and courageous (7 seconds pause)
29. You forgive yourself for all the past mistakes (7 seconds pause)
30. You stay in present and are more mindful (7 seconds pause)
31. You are confident (7 seconds pause)

32. You have high self-esteem (7 seconds pause)
33. You are losing weight every day (7 seconds pause)
34. You are focused on your weight loss journey (7 seconds pause)
35. You pay attention to your food intake (7 seconds pause)
36. You chew your food many times (7 seconds pause)
37. You maintain sleep hygiene (7 seconds pause)
38. You love yourself unconditionally (7 seconds pause)
39. Your body is getting fitter and slimmer (7 seconds pause)
40. You are successful (7 seconds pause)
41. You are confident and motivated (7 seconds pause)
42. You believe in yourself (7 seconds pause)
43. You are good enough (7 seconds pause)
44. You enjoy healthy foods (7 seconds pause)
45. You do pleasurable activities everyday (7 seconds pause)
46. You are intelligent and wise (7 seconds pause)
47. You are lovable, open to receive and give love (7 seconds pause)
48. You enjoy your life (7 seconds pause)
49. You enjoy healthy food (7 seconds pause)
50. You have a beautiful relationship with food and your body (7 seconds pause)
51. You have a lot of love and approval for yourself. (7 seconds pause)
52. You are at peace with yourself in your body, heart and soul. (7 seconds pause)
53. As each day passes, you feel that you are healthier and stronger inside. (7 seconds pause)
54. Every day, you are learning how to love and appreciate your body. (7 seconds pause)
55. Being yourself is the safest way for you to be. (7 seconds pause)
56. You focus on all the good that is happening in your life. (7 seconds pause)
57. It becomes easier and easier for you to trust your body. (7 seconds pause)
58. You can feel your body and mind getting healed. (7 seconds pause)
59. You are choosing to take in breaths of relaxation and breathe out all your stress. (7 seconds pause)
60. Your health and your life are moving in the direction of improvement. (7 seconds pause)
61. A healing white light surrounds you and is protecting you. (7 seconds pause)
62. Your entire food intake is nourishing your body and healing it well. (7 seconds pause)
63. Every baby step you take is getting you closer to your ideal goal weight. (7 seconds pause)

64. You progress comes above any perfection for you. (7 seconds pause)
65. Your intuition is your guiding light and helps you decide what to eat and how to live your life. (7 seconds pause)
66. You are naturally connecting with like-minded people who bring in positivity. (7 seconds pause)
67. It is best for you to let go of your past. Letting go of the past is safe for you now. (7 seconds pause)
68. You can feel the beginning of changes in everything around you. (7 seconds pause)
69. You are now focused, determined and healthy. (7 seconds pause)
70. You choose for yourself to be slim and healthy. (7 seconds pause)
71. You can see new doors opening in your life with a lot of new and exciting things. (7 seconds pause)
72. You have the ability to heal your body. You are healing your body. (7 seconds pause)
73. You can do this and so you are doing this. Your body is healing right now. (7 seconds pause)
74. A higher power is guiding you along your way. (7 seconds pause)
75. You are a strong, energetic person. (7 seconds pause)
76. You choose to see the best in everyone and so do they. (7 seconds pause)
77. You have faith in your ability of self-love. (7 seconds pause)
78. You truly love yourself for however you are. (7 seconds pause)
79. You have accepted and acknowledged your body shape and the beauty hidden in it.
80. You are the creator of your future. (7 seconds pause)
81. You have now moved on from the unhealthy, unhelpful behavioral pattern around food. (7 seconds pause)
82. The choices and decisions you make for yourself are for your higher good. (7 seconds pause)
83. You are no longer holding on to any regrets or guilt about your past food choices. (7 seconds pause)
84. You have accepted your body's shape and you feel blessed for what you have. (7 seconds pause)
85. You have moved farther away from relationships that don't contribute to your betterment. (7 seconds pause)
86. You acknowledge your own greatness. (7 seconds pause)
87. You allow yourself to feel good about being you. (7 seconds pause)
88. You have an acceptance for yourself. (7 seconds pause)
89. You are letting in the qualities of love in your heart. (7 seconds pause)

90. You see your future filled with hope and certainty. (7 seconds pause)
91. You find gratefulness in your heart for your body and all you do for your well-being. (7 seconds pause)
92. You indulge in a healthy amount of exercise on a regular basis. (7 seconds pause)
93. Your body is getting all the nutrients that it requires. (7 seconds pause)
94. You are developing a strong urge to eat food that is nutritious (7 seconds pause)
95. You feel good about yourself. (7 seconds pause)
96. You are on your way to attaining and maintaining your ideal weight. (7 seconds pause)
97. You are a strong, healthy person. (7 seconds pause)
98. You are now peaceful and calm. (7 seconds pause)
99. The Universe has gifted you with your mind, body and soul. (7 seconds pause)
100. Your body is your temple.
101. You love your body and take care of it every single day.. (7 seconds pause)

Waking Up

In a moment, I am going to count you up from 1 to 5, and with each count up, you will slowly and gradually come back to the here and now.

Starting now

At 1...become aware of your breaths

2...start coming up

3...further up

4...all your spiritual, mental, emotional, physical bodies aligned...

5...feel the clothes on your body...eyes open wide awake.

www.ingramcontent.com/pod-product-compliance
Lightning Source LLC
Chambersburg PA
CBHW080626030426
42336CB00018B/3090